Pelvic Ultrasound Imaging

A Case-Based Approach

Pelvic Ultrasound Imaging
A Case-Based Approach

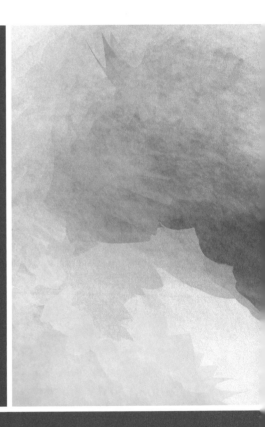

Rebecca Hall, PhD, RDMS, FSDMS

Professor and Clinical Director
Urogynecology Fellow Diagnostic Imaging Program
Department of Obstetrics and Gynecology; Division of Urogynecology
University of New Mexico Health Sciences Center
Albuquerque, New Mexico

ELSEVIER

Elsevier
1600 John F. Kennedy Blvd.
Ste 1600
Philadelphia, PA 19103-2899

PELVIC ULTRASOUND IMAGING

ISBN: 978-0-323-78978-3

Notice

ISBN: 9780323789783

Content Strategist: Nancy Anastasi Duffy
Content Development Manager: Meghan Andress
Content Development Specialist: Deborah Poulson
Publishing Services Manager: Shereen Jameel
Project Manager: Nadhiya Sekar
Design Direction: Bridget Hoette

Printed in the United States of America

Last digit is the print number: 9   8   7   6   5   4   3   2   1

This book is dedicated to our residents and fellows who share our love of diagnostic imaging, and to our patients who give us their trust.

Preface

This book presents a diagnostic pelvic ultrasound imaging workbook that consists of 10 chapters, each with about 40 ultrasound images (figures). A narrative line of directive questions associated with those images is then added to work through individual case assessment—a format that will bring the reader to a diagnostic conclusion. Each case includes one to five figures with the discussion of exam findings, clinical correlation, and interpretation skill development. Detailed steps in 3D instrumentation tools is an addition designed to improve the exam skills of the provider. This approach may serve as a diagnostic imaging primer or a refresher for the advanced practitioner. The reader audience may include urogynecologists and fellows, urologists and fellows, colorectal surgeons and fellows, radiology residents and pelvic imaging specialists, obstetrics/gynecology residents, medical students, and diagnostic medical sonographers specializing in gynecology and/or urogynecology (Gyn/Urogyn).

The workbook concept was derived from years of case review lectures, clinical imaging examinations, and one-on-one didactic sessions with rotating fellows in urogynecology and maternal–fetal medicine, as well as obstetrics/gynecology and radiology residents that resulted in consistent ultrasound imaging and interpretation competency of our trainees. No pelvic imaging case review workbooks have been recently published. While available Gyn/Urogyn ultrasound imaging textbooks are excellent and extremely useful for learners as well as practicing experienced imaging professionals, there is a paucity of pelvic floor images and urogynecology cases typically presented in most texts. This book presents additional considerations for Urogyn case exams.

The format is like a one-on-one oral case review, where a step-by-step image evaluation is done following a clinical ultrasound exam, after which a report is generated. New learners may originally feel overwhelmed with the redundancy of these image assessment questions until they see that a consistent approach broadens their evaluation. The book chapters are written to be progressively more effortful, so the more experienced practitioner may also be challenged as 3D imaging instrumentation is especially highlighted.

The first figure of each chapter will cover a brief general "Topic" or point of interest. The "Topics" are thought to be important considerations in Gyn and Urogyn imaging but are not presented as a specific case; however, the information may be helpful in subsequent chapters. For example, the "Topic" in Chapter 1 is *Semantics in the context of pelvic imaging* and the narrative for Fig. 1 is a brief explanation about the importance of all ultrasound imaging specialists to standardize imaging nomenclature.

The range of diagnostic skills of gynecology, radiology, and urogynecology practitioners is wide. One goal of this workbook is to provide steps to help the new learner perform and assess their own 2D and 3D diagnostic imaging cases in a standard way. For those who may not have one-on-one case development available but desire to learn how diagnostic imaging tools can increase their image understanding, this case-based approach serves as a learning tool so that discussions with the imaging consultants to whom they refer their patients can be improved.

This book presents cases to the reader the way a clinical day unfolds—varied and unrelated to the last case—instead of a pathology-based approach such as "adnexal mass," where similar examples of the same abnormality are consecutively presented. There are no prescribed selected topics or chapter titles in the Table of Contents. This way, the reader can approach each case's findings without diagnostic bias. Individual case images (figures) and narrative questions are followed by the answers at the back of the book. The e-book figures and narrative questions are followed by accessible answers with a designated keystroke button.

Examples of common gynecology cases referred to diagnostic imaging laboratories are included, such as ovarian hemorrhagic corpus luteum and endometrial polyps. More uncommon gynecology cases are also presented, such as ovarian neoplasms. Nearly half of this book is made up of urogynecology cases that include common as well as more uncommon pathologies, such as rectal vaginal fistula, rectal prolapse, and mesh assessment.

Consistent reporting, by highlighting the importance to "describe, describe, describe," is emphasized in summarizing diagnostic imaging pathologies. The diagnostician looks globally, then at details, when assessing ultrasound exam images. If more specifics are desired, especially if 3D volume sets have been acquired, additional instrumentation steps may provide ways to improve diagnostic appraisal.

There are two Appendices:

- Appendix 1 includes a single page of Abbreviations used throughout the book.
- Appendix 2 includes reporting templates that providers may want to incorporate into their practice to standardize their imaging center's reports.

I sincerely hope that these cases will be helpful in pelvic diagnostic ultrasound performance and interpretation skill development.

I would like to thank Jim Merritt, Elsevier's Executive Content Strategist, and Nancy Duffy, my Elsevier Ob/Gyn Portfolio Consultant, my Content Development Specialist, Deborah Poulson, and my Project Manager, Nadhiya Sekar, for their gentle guidance and support in actualizing this workbook project. I also appreciate my Contributing Author, Dr. Lieschen Quiroz, for her invaluable input in the development of the book format and especially her expertise in the discussion of 3D biplane imaging of the pelvic floor. Sincere acknowledgment and recognition go to my Associate Editor, Dr. Peter Jeppson, whose command of medical literature afforded such a careful and thoughtful review of the workbook. Special thanks also to the artist, Rob Bathurst, who so carefully created the anatomic drawings in the same thoughtful way he has approached everything in life, which I know, because he is my oldest son.

Rebecca Hall

Author:
Rebecca Hall, PhD, RDMS, FSDMS
Professor and Clinical Director
Urogynecology Fellow Diagnostic Imaging
Department of Obstetrics and Gynecology; Division of Urogynecology
University of New Mexico Health Sciences Center
Albuquerque, NM, USA

Contributing Author:
Lieschen Quiroz, MD
Associate Professor
Section Chief, Division of Female Pelvic Medicine and Reconstructive Surgery
Department of Obstetrics and Gynecology
University of Oklahoma Health Sciences Center
Oklahoma, OK, USA

Associate Editor:
Peter Jeppson, MD
Associate Professor
Section Chief; Division of Female Pelvic Medicine and Reconstructive Surgery
Department of Obstetrics and Gynecology
University of New Mexico Health Sciences Center
Albuquerque, NM, USA

How Each Chapter Begins

Each chapter in this workbook begins with a brief general topic point of interest. The topics are thought to be important considerations in Gynecologic/Urogynecologic imaging but are not presented in any specific order. No questions are asked of the reader, but the information may be helpful in subsequent cases.

LIST OF TOPICS

Chapter 1: Semantics in the context of pelvic imaging
Chapter 2: How Doppler is used in this workbook
Chapter 3: Approach to exam assessment
Chapter 4: Basic 3D instrumentation
Chapter 5: Normal endoanal 3D image of the distal internal and external anal sphincter
Chapter 6: Tomographic ultrasound imaging of the normal transperineal anal sphincter complex 3D volume set
Chapter 7: Tomographic ultrasound imaging of the abnormal transperineal anal sphincter complex 3D volume set
Chapter 8: "Read" zoom versus "Write" zoom
Chapter 9: Information on the 3D volume set screen is abundant
Chapter 10: Anal sphincter complex Color Power Doppler pulse repetition frequency setting changes

Case Reviews

Video Contents

Case Reviews 1–18

Outline

Each chapter in this workbook will begin with a brief general Topic point of interest. Diagnostic imaging topics are an important aspect of gynecology and urogynecology and are presented throughout the book in no specific order. No questions are asked of the Learner, but the information may be helpful in subsequent cases.

TOPIC 1, FIGURE 1

1. Fig. 1. Topic: Semantics in the context of pelvic imaging

   If a transducer is placed in the vagina, the exam is commonly referred to as "transvaginal" when, in fact, it is "endovaginal" or from within. We will use the term "endocavitary," "endovaginal," or "endorectal" in our case discussions. In this workbook, when referring to the placement of the transducer, the prefix "trans" implies "through" a structure, whereas the prefix "endo" implies "from within" a structure. The term "transperineal" is appropriate to use for an exam because the transducer is placed at the perineum through which sound waves are propagated to assess the pelvic floor structures.

   Semantics in the context of pelvic imaging matters to the patient. In this workbook, the term "transducer" is used as opposed to the term "probe" for instrumentation description. Furthermore, the term "transducer" is also used for the ultrasound examination instrument when discussing findings to our patients, as well as in our reporting. When a patient hears the examiner talk about the exam "probe," for example, during an anal sphincter complex exam, it is our contention that what they hear is, "I'm going to probe your rectum now."

   We recognize that the manufacturing vendors making the transducer may call the housing unit the "probe" and the source component that produces the ultrasound the "transducer," but we will, nevertheless, use the term "transducer" throughout this workbook and not the term "probe."

> **Case Review: Chapter 1**
> **Topic: Semantics in the context of pelvic imaging: "Transvaginal" versus "Endovaginal"**
> **and**
> **"Transducer" versus "Probe"**

Fig. 1

CASE 1, FIGURES 2 AND 3

2. Figs. 2 and 3 are endovaginal (EV) images of a 2D midline (ML) sagittal uterus and a transverse mid-uterus. The directional relationship of the EV transducer to the patient's perineum on the screen is consistent, but can be consistent, but can be confusing to the learner, especially in the presence of pathology. To the learner it seems logical that if the transducer is placed on the thyroid, for example, the transducer would be at the top of the screen and the anterior aspect of the thyroid would be under the transducer on the image. If the transabdominal transducer is placed at the anterior pelvis

on an anteverted uterus, for example, the transducer would be at the top of the screen and the anterior aspect of the uterus would be under the transducer on the screen.

This may not be so apparent when pathology is found on a gynecologic EV ultrasound exam or when performing transperineal pelvic floor imaging. In the United States, the standard is that wherever the transducer is, the anatomy under the transducer is placed at the top of the screen. In other countries, the standard may be reversed. Since the transducer is in the vagina, it is located inferior relative to the patient's body. So, if the transducer is in the vagina and the patient were to stand upright, the transducer would be angled toward the floor, which is inferior to HER BODY, but the transducer would still be at the top of the screen.

Additionally, the standard for the left side of the screen on the EV sagittal plane is anterior and the right side is posterior. For the transverse plane, when the transducer is turned 90 degrees to the patient's right side by standard (left on the examiner's hand), the patient's right side is on the left side of the image, as if one is looking up the anatomy from her feet toward her head.

This assumes the examiner is holding the transducer correctly. All transducers have a notch on the top of the handle, so by touching that aspect of the transducer with the gloved hand before placing the transducer, the examiner will see the moving fingertip on the screen location before placement. If, for example, you are in a transverse plane and you angle to the patient's right side, what is right will come into view. This becomes second nature in endovaginal imaging but is important to do correctly. Otherwise, in the presence of pathology, location of findings may be completely backward.

a. In Figs. 2 and 3, in what direction **on the patient** is the top of the screen for both planes (sagittal and transverse)? _____
b. In what position is the uterus—anteverted, neutral, or retroverted? _____
c. Is the uterus anteflexed, retroflexed, or neither? _____

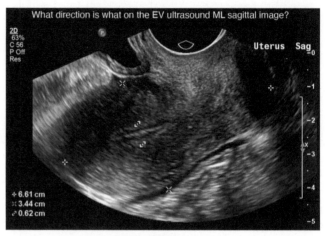

Fig. 2

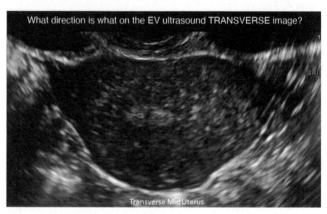

Fig. 3

CASE 2, FIGURES 4 AND 5

3. Figs. 4 and 5 are labeled with correct directional locations. To what aspect of the uterus in each plane is the gold arrow pointing—anterior or posterior?
    a. Fig. 4 _____
    b. Fig. 5 _____

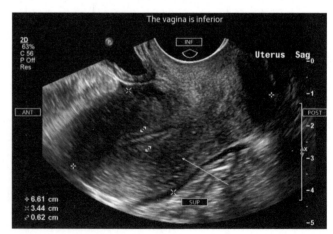

Fig. 4

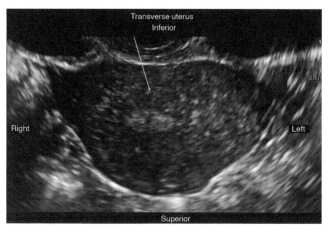

Fig. 5

CASE 3, FIGURES 6–10

4. Fig. 6 is a transperineal 3D volume set of a normal urethra. When a volume is made, it is easy to forget that much more anatomic information is available to assess than what is seen on the screen. The 3D rendered image (screen bottom right) can be removed, as in this case. Image A (see red arrow) is always the original sweep plane and, in this case, is a midsagittal plane. If only a 2D midline sagittal image was done, it would look exactly the same as the A plane image.

   The degree of sweep, which is determined by the examiner, was made with an arbitrary 75-degree sweep angle to capture the entire adjacent lateral anatomy.

   The sweep speed (also determined by the examiner) was set at the slowest option to maximize the resolution. Contrarily, if the sweep speed is set too high, the image resolution will decrease.

   Look at the small dot on all three images. That dot, called the center reference point (CRP), or, alternatively, the axis center point, is the center of the anatomic sweep volume and can be moved on any plane by the examiner or post exam at a workstation. When it is moved on one plane cutting through the anatomic volume, it will move on all three planes in that same direction; therefore, one can parallel shift through the entire volume in any plane.

   Note that the white dot on the A plane is at the anterior aspect of the mid-urethra (yellow arrow).

Figs. 7 and 8 demonstrate slices through the original A plane in orthogonal B and C planes; therefore, the B plane is coronal to the urethral A plane at that dot (yellow line, as if you are looking anteriorly from behind the urethra) and the C plane is axial to the urethral cut through the A plane at that dot (faint blue, as if you are looking from one side to the other on the A plane). Sometimes, planes get confusing. It is always a good idea to distinguish any cut as a plane relative to the body versus the specific anatomy. It feels redundant to spend so much time on this at first when it is normal anatomy, but it pays off when there is pathology.

   a. On the A plane, at what direction on the patient's body is the top of the screen? _____
   b. On the B plane, at what direction on the patient's body is the top of the screen? _____
   c. On the C plane, at what direction on the patient's body is the bottom of the screen? _____
   d. On the A plane, at what direction on the patient's body is the bottom of the screen? _____
   e. On the B plane, at what direction on the patient's body is the bottom of the screen? _____
   f. On the A plane, at what direction on the patient's body is the left of the screen? _____
   g. On the B plane, at what direction on the patient's body is the left of the screen? _____

5. Transperineal 3D imaging greatly enhances mesh placement confidence, and manipulation of the 3D volume set can confirm and augment 2D pelvic floor findings. Fig. 9 goes back to the original 3D volume sweep. With the top of the screen as inferior, the red lines are placed at distal (screen top), mid and proximal aspects of the urethra.

   The mid-urethra is the ideal location for mesh placement. Visualization of the mesh on the A plane is seen as a hyperechoic focus posterior to the mid-urethra (yellow arrow), as if the mesh is coming at you, so it is seen on end; therefore, the C plane, created by the cut at the CRP dot on the A plane will show the side-to-side axial mid-urethra image behind which is the mesh. Why do we not see any mesh on the B plane? Fig. 10 demonstrates how the C plane can be pulled out of the volume set and rotated on the Z-axis to better present the midlevel suburethral mesh.

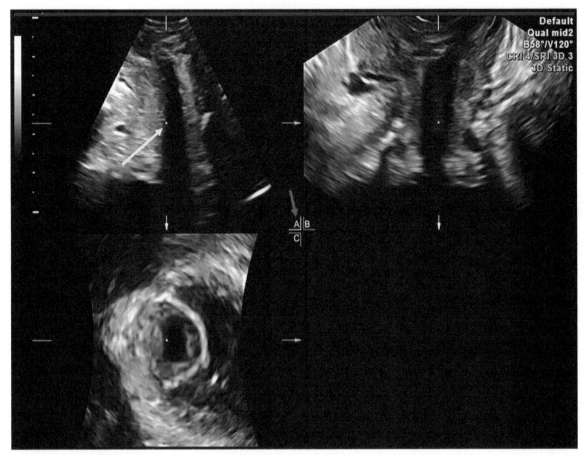

Fig. 6

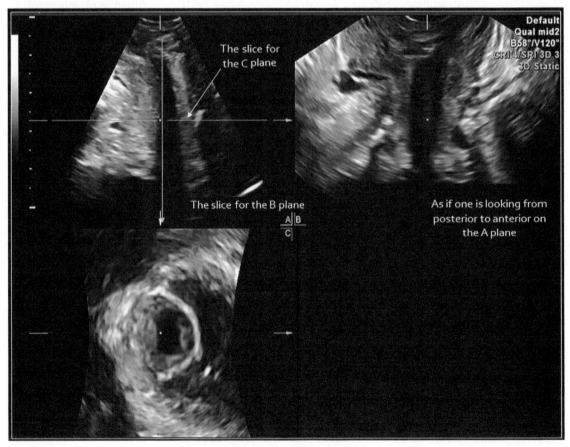

Fig. 7

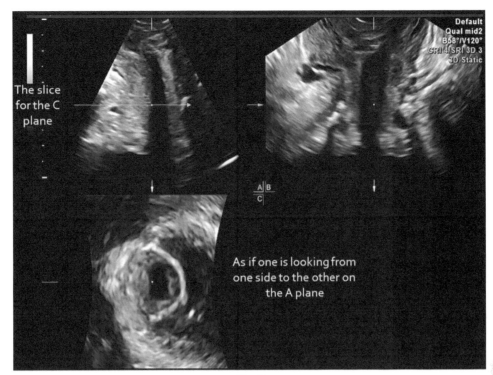

Fig. 8

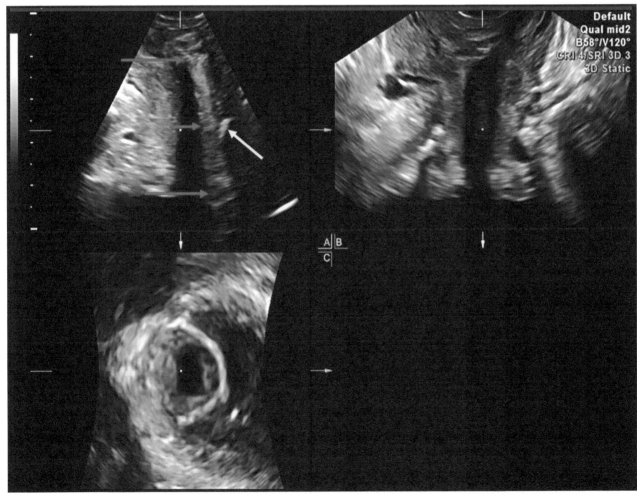

Fig. 9

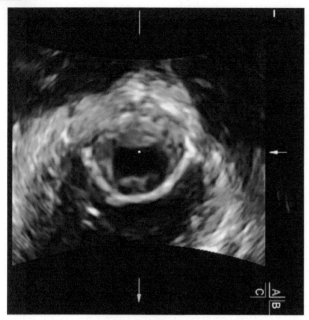

Fig. 10

CASE 4, FIGURE 11

6. Fig. 11 is an EV midsagittal image of a nulliparous uterus. The patient's last menstrual period (LMP) was 6 days ago. In what direction on the patient should the transducer handle be directed to see the entire uterine fundus? _____

7. The endometrium demonstrates several subtle thin layers on the midsagittal plane which can demonstrate anatomic changes in appearance throughout the endometrial cycle. At what phase of the cycle is the endometrium—proliferative or secretory? _____

8. To what is the letter "d" pointing? _____

9. In every image, there is a focal zone displayed by a carrot mark or a line of range along the side of the caliper markings where a convergence of the transducer's lines of sight is located. The focal zone is moved throughout the exam to the area of interest so that the image is most focused there. Is the focal zone (green arrow) placed at the most optimal level to assess the endometrium? _____

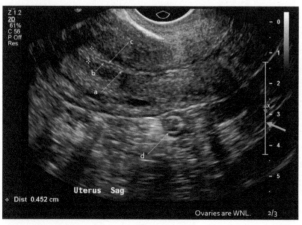

Fig. 11

CASE 5, FIGURE 12

10. Fig. 12. In what position is this midsagittal image of a uterus? _____

11. What segment of the uterus is the "A" location? _____

12. In what direction on the patient is the "B" location? _____

13. In what direction on the patient is the "C" location? _____

14. In what direction on the patient is the "D" location? _____

15. In what direction on the patient is the "E" location? _____

16. In what direction on the patient should the transducer be moved to better see the posterior cul-de-sac free fluid (*)? _____

17. At what phase of the cycle is the endometrium? _____

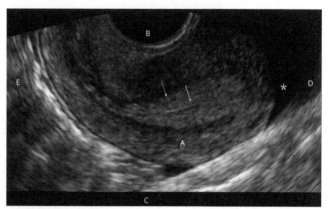

Fig. 12

CASE 6, FIGURES 13 AND 14

18. Figs. 13 and 14 demonstrate a 3D volume set of a uterus with a sagittal original sweep acquisition (A) plane. Note the center reference points on the three orthogonal planes. Another important tool to specify areas of interest is the dotted green line of reference (LOR). The LOR, which is operator dependent, is moved on the A and B planes to any level within the volume; in this case, it is just above the endometrium to 3D render the endometrium in Fig. 14.

If the LOR is not brought down to the endometrium, the anterior myometrium would be 3D rendered and the endometrium would not be seen. It would still be in the volume set but below the myometrium under the higher LOR.

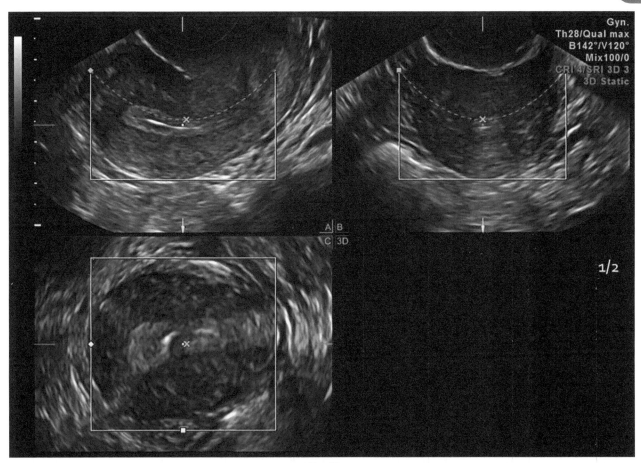

Fig. 13

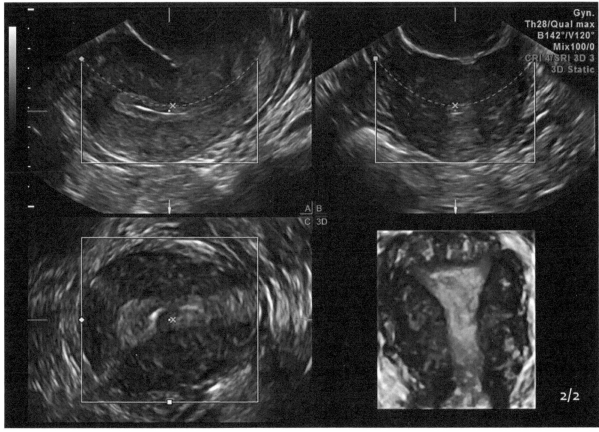

Fig. 14

CASE 7, FIGURE 15

Fig. 15 is a 3D volume set of the uterus performed to assess correct placement of a recently placed Essure coil on a patient with new onset of postoperative pelvic pain. The center reference point (CRP) location is completely operator dependent and will alter all images with every move through the area of interest on the entire volume set.

There are three knobs on ultrasound 3D system control panels that are labeled X, Y, and Z. Each is a rotary control to allow rotation of the anatomy through any 3D volume set by rotating on any axis in order to display any desired plane within the volume. Turning the X knob would rotate the planes by slicing through the volume as if shaking it "yes." Turning the Y knob would rotate the planes by slicing through the volume as if shaking it "no." Turning the Z knob would rotate the plane as if "doing a cartwheel." So, in this case, by rotating the "Y"-axis, the left coil would "stretch out" as seen on the added rotated rendered image. On which side of the uterus is the CRP placed in the images? _____

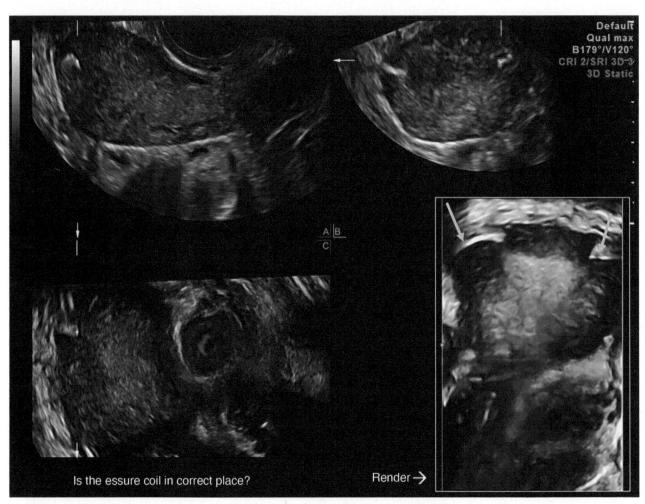

Fig. 15

CASE 8, FIGURES 16 AND 17

19. Fig. 16 is a transperineal rotated upright C plane image of the urethra behind which is a suburethral sling from a transperineal 3D volume of the urethra complex using a 5–9 MHz EV transducer. The patient presented with postoperative urethral sling placement pain. On which side of the image is the patient's right side? _____

20. Can one tell from this single image if the sling is at the mid-urethral level? (Does seeing the mesh posterior to the urethra imply the appropriate location?)

    a. Yes _____

    b. No _____

    c. Cannot tell _____

21. Fig. 17 demonstrates the entire 3D volume set and is crucial to assess when the mesh placement, relative to surrounding anatomy, is the reason for the exam. The echogenic linear focus on the A plane is seen posterior to the urethra, as if the focus is coming toward you on end. Of note, the urethra, which

is typically well visualized, is not well seen along the entire sagittal image with noted angulation of the contour. The gold arrows point to the distal, mid, and proximal levels (screen top to bottom).

The center reference point (CRP) has been placed on the mesh on the A plane (midsagittal of the mesh); therefore, the B plane (coronal of the mesh) and the C plane (transverse or axial of the mesh) demonstrate the CRP in a central location along the posterior edge of the mesh.

Is the mesh located at the mid-urethra? _____

22. Note that the 3D rendered image demonstrates an additional echogenic focus that was consistently seen throughout the exam (red arrow). Try to assess the location of this urethral focus. Our report is provided in the Answer Key.

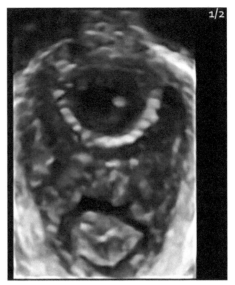

Fig. 16

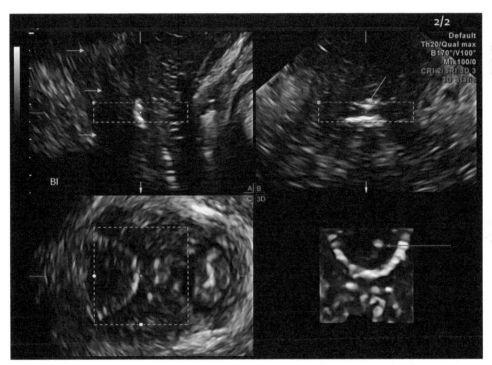

Fig. 17

CASE 9, FIGURE 18

23. Fig. 18 demonstrates a 3D rendered image of the uterus with an intrauterine device recently placed centrally within the endometrial cavity. Identify the following labeled structures:

   a. _____
   b. _____
   c. _____
   d. _____

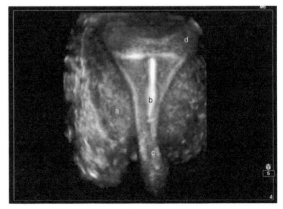

Fig. 18

CASE 10, FIGURES 19–21

24. Figs. 19–21 demonstrate uterine sagittal and transverse images of a 40-year-old primiparous patient with known leiomyomata of various echogenic patterns.

   Is the uterus small, normal, or enlarged in size? _____

25. In what position [anteverted (AV), retroverted (RV), anteflexed (AF), retroflexed (RF)] is the uterus?
   a. AV, AF
   b. AV
   c. RV
   d. RV, RF

26. Fig. 19. The red arrow is placed on the basal layer, the white arrow is placed on the functional layer, and the green arrow is placed on the apposing walls of the endometrial cavity. In what phase of the menstrual cycle is the endometrium?
   a. Post menses
   b. Early proliferative phase
   c. Proliferative phase
   d. Mid-cycle
   e. Secretory phase

27. Which of the following would best describe the endometrium?
   a. The endometrium appears elevated at the lower uterine segment by a posterior segment myomatous lesion.
   b. The endometrium appears elevated at the mid-uterine segment by posterior segment myomatous lesions.
   c. The endometrium appears elevated at the mid-uterine segment by an anterior submucosal myomatous lesion.
   d. The endometrium appears elevated at the mid-fundal endometrial segment by multiple posterior/fundal myomatous lesions.

28. The uterus is heterogeneous in echo pattern. Improved visualization of the overall echo pattern can be achieved by choosing from several chroma options without changing any of the sonographic information, as shown in Figs. 20 and 21. Although a single myomatous lesion is measured, the more you look at the overall pattern, the more lesions you see throughout the myometrium. The more you look, the more you see. Which differential diagnosis is *incorrect*?
   a. Diffuse leiomyomata
   b. Intramural leiomyomata
   c. Submucosal leiomyomata
   d. Subserosal leiomyomata

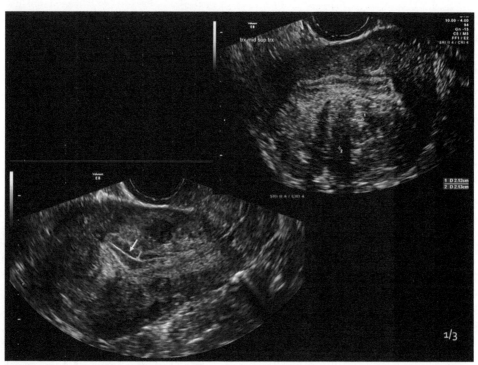

Fig. 19

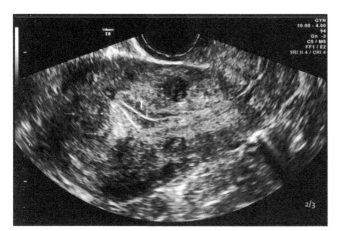

Fig. 20

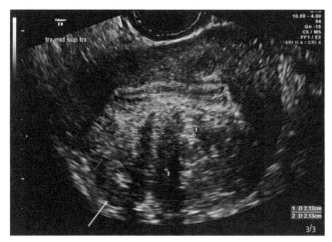

Fig. 21

CASE 11, FIGURES 22–24

29. Figs. 22–23 demonstrate EV images of the right ovary of a patient with sudden onset of right lower quadrant pain. The left ovary and uterus appear within normal limits in size and echo pattern and are not shown here. The ovary, measuring approximately 3.3 × 2.6 × 3.5 cm, contains a complex primarily cystic appearing mass with an irregular contoured hyperechoic subcomponent. Note that the hyperechoic area appears to be in a different location on the transverse cut compared with the sagittal cut of the ovary.
   a. In the transverse plane, in what directions on her body are the labels in Fig. 22:
      A _____
      B _____
      C _____
      D _____
   b. In the sagittal plane, in what directions on her body are the labels in Fig. 23:
      A _____
      B _____
      C _____
      D _____

30. Fig. 24 labels the correct directions for each plane. Understanding the directional locations for each plane is significant in diagnostic criteria and confidence of diagnosis. Since the patient is lying supine for the exam and as the echogenic aspect is lying inferiorly and posteriorly, one can assume that it is dependent. When the patient was rotated on the table to a right lateral decubitus position, the hyperechoic subcomponent began to shift in position. What is the most likely etiology? _____

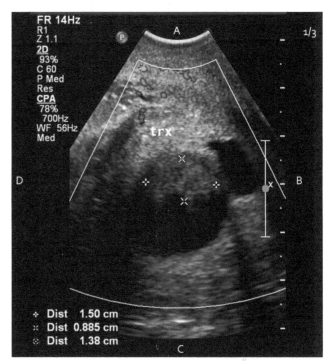

Fig. 22

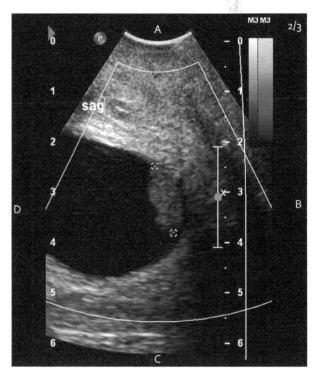

Fig. 23

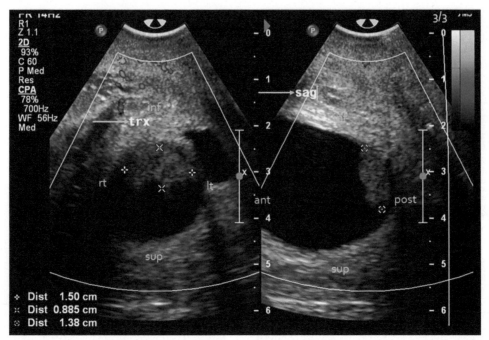

Fig. 24

CASE 12, FIGURES 25–27

31. Figs. 25–27 represent images using a 4–8 MHz EV transducer for a pelvic exam in a 47-year-old following her annual exam, referred when the provider noted right adnexal fullness. The patient's last menstrual period was 7 days ago.

    The normal ovary measures approximately 1 × 2 × 3 cm. This may change through the cycle as follicles and a corpus luteum form, grow, and resolve. What is the approximate size of each ovary? Be sure to note that the measurement calipers scales are different in Figs. 25 and 26.

  a. Fig. 25. Right ovary _____
  b. Fig. 26. Left ovary _____
  c. Do the ovaries demonstrate a normal echo pattern? _____

32. Do both ovaries have normal contour?
  a. Right ovary _____
  b. Left ovary _____

33. Do both ovaries demonstrate normal appearing follicles?
  a. Right ovary _____
  b. Left ovary _____

34. Figs. 26 and 27. Color Power Doppler can be used to assess the presence of global vascularity. As is seen here, there is a single color applied to the vessels present, which is a qualitative identification of vascularity but no directional or velocity of flow information. Does the Color Power Doppler pattern appear within normal limits of the left ovary? _____

35. Does the Doppler resistive index (RI) add to, not affect, or reduce your concern for a malignant outcome? _____

36. The exam report should contain a detailed description of all the above for this abnormal appearance. Findings suggest the presence of:
  a. Simple cyst
  b. Hemorrhagic corpus luteum
  c. Neoplasm
  d. Dermoid

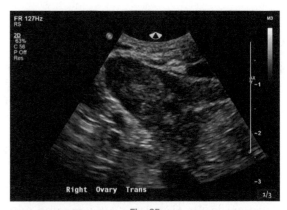

Fig. 25

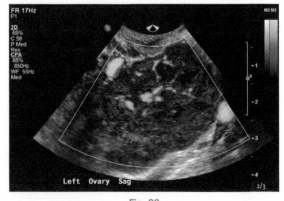

Fig. 26

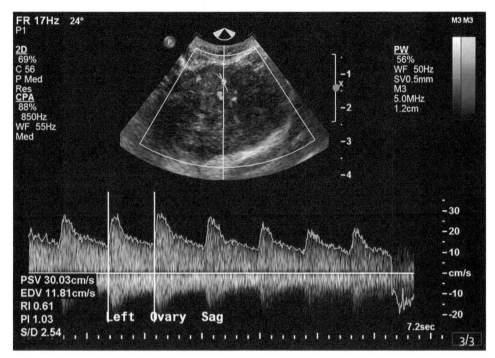

Fig. 27

CASE 13, FIGURE 28

37. Fig. 28 demonstrates a transperineal 3D volume set of the anal sphincter complex using a 5–9 MHz EV transducer to assess the puboviceralis muscle (PVM) complex. In what plane is the 3D sweep made, as seen in the A image? _____

38. At what aspect of the vagina in all three orthogonal planes is the center reference point (CRP) seen? _____

39. On what plane would the operator move the CRP to assess the urethra since it is in the volume sweep? _____

40. With the (green) line of reference brought down to the CRP on the A plane, the rendered image demonstrates the PVM complex. Is there evidence of avulsion? _____

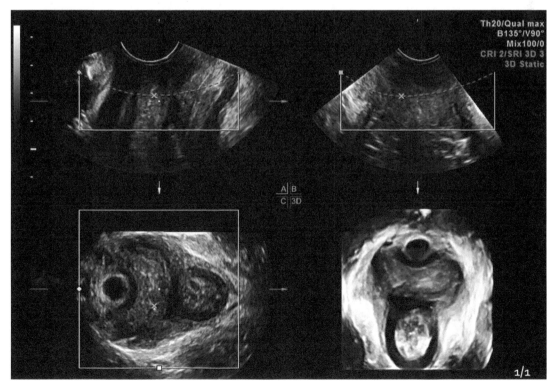

Fig. 28

CASE 14, FIGURES 29–31

41. Figs. 29 and 30 demonstrate transverse images of the mid- and lower uterine segment and Fig. 31 is a parasagittal image of the peripheral uterine vasculature in a 38-year-old patient with chronic central pelvic pain, described as "aching." The exam was performed using a 5–9 MHz EV transducer. The ovaries appear normal and are not presented here.

Even without the color Doppler application, there is clear evidence of diffuse abnormally prominent vascularity measuring 6 mm (gold line). Fig. 31 demonstrates how the uterine vasculature changed with the patient performing a Valsalva maneuver. Use of Doppler to demonstrate retrograde flow may be evident with Doppler color flow or Doppler spectral waveform but is not performed here.

   a. What is the typical anteroposterior diameter of the ovarian venous vessels? _____
   b. Does the diameter of the pelvic vascularity remain the same, decrease, or increase with Valsalva? _____
   c. The noticeable diffuse uterine peripheral vessels are indicative of what diagnosis? _____
   d. Is this patient more likely to be nulliparous or multiparous? _____

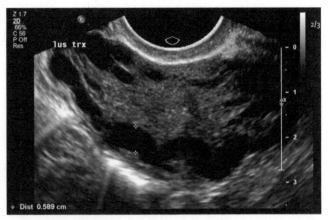

Fig. 29

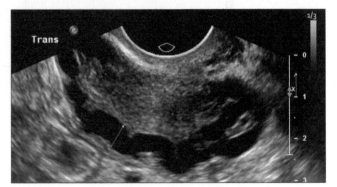

Fig. 30

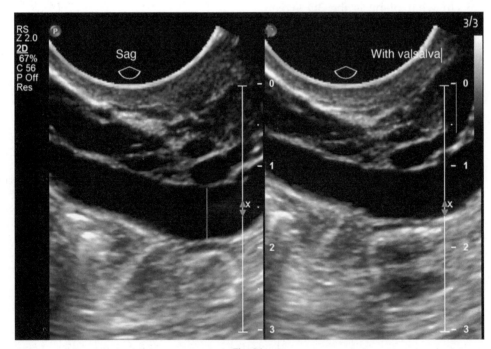

Fig. 31

CASE 15, FIGURES 32 AND 33

42. Figs. 32 and 33 are sagittal and transverse images of a 24-year-old woman with a history of infertility and menorrhagia, or abnormal uterine bleeding, who is on day 8 of her cycle.

    In what position is the uterus? _____

43. A normal endometrium on day 8 would not have the same appearance as is seen in Figs. 32 and 33. Note that the thin hyperechoic endometrial lining representing the basal endometrium (gold arrow) entirely envelops a thin hypoechoic layer representing the functional layer that entirely envelops a smooth-walled homogeneous hyperechoic central endometrial cavity structure. In what phase of the menstrual cycle does this endometrium appearance confirm?
    a. Post menses
    b. Early proliferative phase
    c. Proliferative phase
    d. Mid-cycle
    e. Secretory phase

44. Describe the central mass in terms of size. _____

45. Determining whether the *origin* of this central lesion is endometrial or uterine in nature is crucial to diagnostic confidence and clinical planning. How does the color Doppler pattern (Fig. 33; color image is black and white) help determine the diagnosis? _____

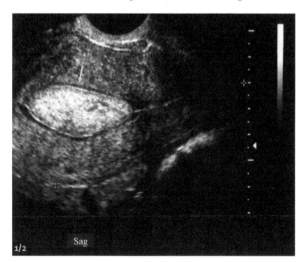

Fig. 32

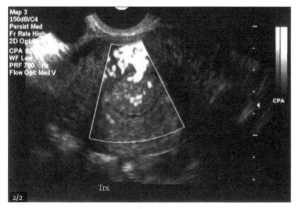

Fig. 33

CASE 16, FIGURES 34–36

46. Figs. 34–36 are endometrial cuts from three separate cases referred for abnormal uterine bleeding with heavy menses as the presenting symptom. Sonohysterography was performed in all three cases with sterile saline injected into the endometrial cavity. The injected fluid can be infused through various types of catheters. In these cases, 10 cc of sterile bacteriostatic water was injected through a 5-Fr Goldstein catheter to expand the endometrium and better delineate the cavity, which may have merely appeared to have an irregular thickened lining prior to the procedure. Endometrial measurements should be included in all exams prior to a sonohysterography procedure.
    a. What intracavity finding do all three cases demonstrate? _____
    b. Which of the cases demonstrates a single lesion? _____
    c. How does Color Power Doppler enhance diagnostic confidence in Fig. 35? _____
    d. The best time to perform a sonohysterogram is just post menses so that the sloughed off functional layer leaves the thin basal endometrial layer. Do these procedure images suggest that the timing for the procedure was appropriate? _____
    e. Does the Color Power Doppler demonstrate any velocity values on the image (Fig. 36)? _____
    f. Fig. 36. Does the color Doppler application appear to be adjusted correctly to visualize the lowest flow vasculature? _____

47. Which one of the following procedural descriptions best describes Fig. 36 findings?

    Under sterile conditions and with patient consent, a sonohysterogram was performed using a 5-Fr Goldstein catheter and 10 cc of sterile bacteriostatic water was infused without incident.

    Findings within the cavity include the following:
    a. An endometrial lesion was visualized and appears hyperechoic compared with the adjacent myometrium. Color Doppler reveals feeder vessels entering into the central lesion. The finding is consistent with an endometrial polyp.
    b. Multiple endometrial lesions were visualized. The echo pattern of lesions is isoechoic to myometrium. Color Doppler reveals peripheral concentric flow pattern. Findings are consistent with submucosal leiomyomata.
    c. Multiple endometrial lesions at the anterior and posterior endometrial segments were visualized and appear isoechoic compared with the adjacent endometrium. Color Doppler reveals feeder vessels entering into all the lesions. Findings are consistent with endometrial polyps.

d. An endometrial lesion at the anterior lining is visualized and appears hyperechoic compared with the adjacent myometrium. Color Doppler reveals feeder vessels entering into the lesion.

Additionally, there are several myomatous lesions seen within the endometrium originating from the posterior endometrial–myometrial interface. The echo pattern of lesions is isoechoic to myometrium. Color Doppler reveals peripheral concentric flow pattern of each lesion. Findings are consistent with concomitant endometrial polyps and submucosal leiomyomata.

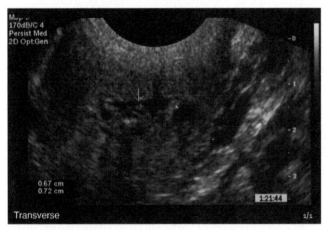

Fig. 34

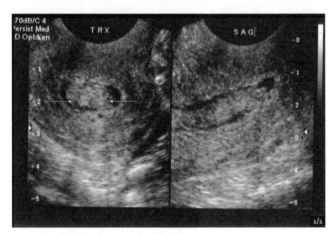

Fig. 35

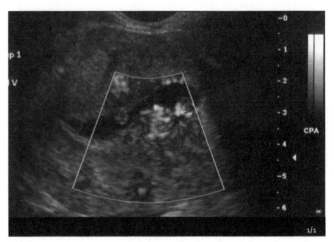

Fig. 36

CASE 17, FIGURES 37 AND 38

48. Figs. 37 and 38 demonstrate how 3D can enhance the assessment of a paraovarian structure that is perceived to be folded over itself. In this case, an anechoic tortuous structure was found incidentally in a 33-year-old woman with bilateral normal ovaries. Once a 3D volume set was made, rotation of the X, Y, and Z axes on the exam control panel was made to elongate any curved structure. OMNI tracing, done by the examiner either during the exam or post exam at a 3D workstation, can then be drawn through the curves of the serpiginous anechoic structure.

The image will elongate the curves as if the "bent" components are "stretched out" as seen on the right half of Figs. 37 and 38 (top).

In this kind of case, each is shown to be all one structure, stretched out and then measured to elicit a more realistic length assessment. 3D imaging has correlative calipers to 2D that are also along the side of images. Fig. 38 (bottom screen right) demonstrates the 3D rendered image of the structure as if seen on end. The planes can be parallel shifted through the entire contiguous length. Though the 2D appearance could quite easily result in the same diagnosis, it is another example of how 3D imaging can easily enhance the diagnostic findings. What is the sonographic diagnosis? _____

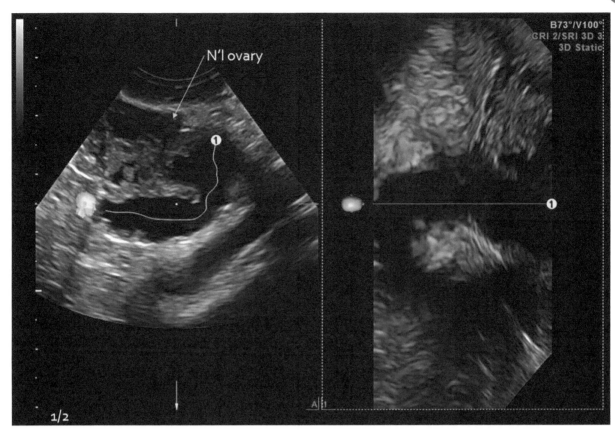

N'l ovary

Fig. 37

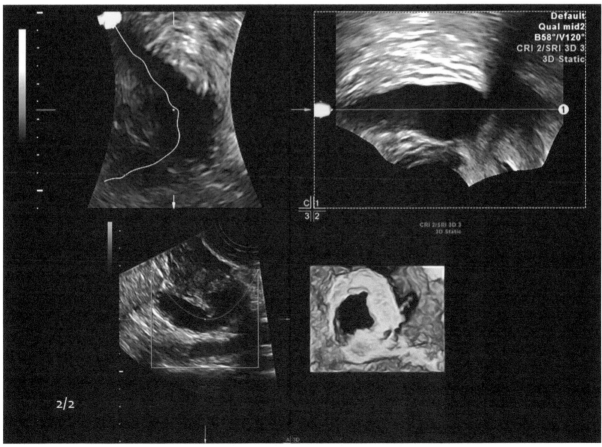

Fig. 38

CASE 18, FIGURES 39 AND 40

49. Figs. 39 and 40 demonstrate a 3D volume set of the normal uterus of a 31-year-old woman.

    In what plane is the initial 3D sweep made? _____

50. Which of the following is the correct position [anteverted (AV), retroverted (RV), neutral, anteflexed (AF), retroflexed (RF)] of the uterus?
    a. AV, AF
    b. AV, RF
    c. Neutral
    d. RV
    e. RV, RF
    f. RV, AF

    Because the uterus is RV, the 3D-rendered image will be upside down by conventional 3D formatting but can be rotated 180 degrees on the Z-axis to see it in the more intuitive typical rendered upright appearance, as seen in Fig. 40.

Note that there appears to be a thin "covering" over the right mid-uterine/cornua segment (white arrow). This is not an artifact, but real anatomy on the image because the green line of reference (LOR) on the 3D volume set (Fig. 39) does not come all the way down to the fundal end of the endometrium (arrows), leaving some myometrium on the image.

If the A plane uterine fundus (screen right) had been rotated on the Z-axis toward the top of the screen, and the LOR brought down ever so slightly, the image would have been cleared up. This seems a little frivolous for a normal 3D volume set of a normal uterus, but awareness of that LOR may prevent unnecessary misdiagnosis, especially in the presence of pathology. If one uses the available tools for normal exams, it will not be so difficult when the anatomy is abnormal when confidence in 3D manipulation needs to be present.

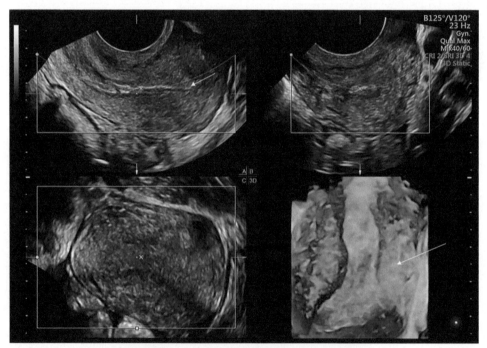

Fig. 39

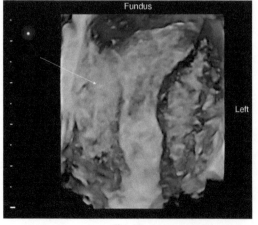

Fig. 40

Case Reviews 19–35

2

TOPIC 2, FIGURE 41

1. Fig. 41. Topic: How Doppler Is Used in This Workbook

   Doppler assessment of vasculature in pelvic diagnostic imaging is common though there are broad variations in knobology settings among ultrasound systems. The examiner should optimize the Doppler settings to ensure that the real vessels are seen, especially in the presence of suspected abnormal vascularization. It is equally important to demonstrate "real" low-velocity vascularization.

   The examiner can choose Color Power Doppler (screen bottom left), color Doppler color flow (screen top left), or Doppler spectral waveform (screen right). Color power Doppler is a qualitative setting, picking up non-directional global vascularity, although some ultrasound systems can also demonstrate blood flow direction with Color Power. Doppler color flow depicts vascularity, with an assigned blue or red pixel application based on mean flow velocity of blood vessels at each location, and identifies flow direction. In the standard setting, red indicates blood flow toward the transducer and blue indicates blood flow away from the transducer.

   In pelvic imaging, it generally does not matter which direction the blood flow is traveling; therefore, the use of Color Power Doppler is reasonable. If Color power Doppler is turned on and no flow within the tissue is seen on the screen, it does not usually indicate absence of flow. It means that the default pulse repetition frequency (PRF) setting for that gynecologic exam may be set too high. PRF is the number of pulses of a repeating signal in a specific time unit, normally measured in pulses per second. On turning down the PRF knob too low, the flow increases until the whole screen "blushes" with diffuse, falsely colored pixels. At this point, the PRF can be turned back up in small increments until the blush disappears and real flow remains. If actual flow velocity of a vessel is needed, Doppler Spectral Waveform analysis of the desired vessels can be subsequently performed to obtain Doppler indices comparing the velocities during systole and diastole.

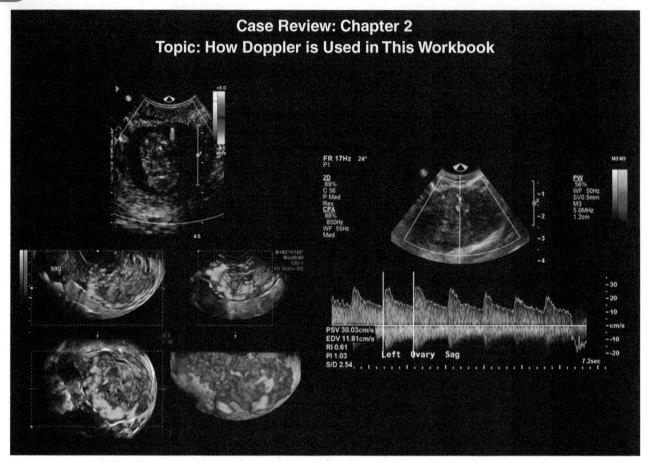

Fig. 41

CASE 19, FIGURE 42

2. Fig. 42 includes two transperineal transverse (axial) cuts of the internal anal sphincter (IAS) surrounding the central mucosa (CM) at the mid-level of the anal sphincter complex (ASC) using a 4–8 MHz endovaginal (EV) transducer in a postpartum patient with perineal pain. If the frequency of the EV transducer was higher, the image resolution would be better, but the depth of penetration would be reduced. Every imaging center will have different transducers available to perform the exam. The examiner should choose the transducer with the highest frequency to optimize the resolution without compromising the depth of visualized anatomy.

The IAS is not intact and there is elevation of the CM toward the defect. In terms of a clock, where would you describe the IAS disruption (red arrows) at the screen top image? _____

3. In a vaginal delivery tear (Fig. 42), postpartum inflammation of the perineum is anticipated, which would demonstrate increased vascularity.

Doppler Color Power was performed in the bottom right image of Fig. 42 to demonstrate the presumed evidence of a perianal inflammatory process in this patient. As described in Fig. 41 Topic

comment above, when a gynecologic setting is initiated at the beginning of a gynecology exam, appreciate that the manufacturer's presets are global settings to be used as a starting point for the exam. All vessels present will not automatically "light up" by merely turning on the Doppler Color Power of blood flow. Turning up the overall "gain" knob increases the echogenicity of all aspects of the screen but is not related to improving visualization of small inflamed blood vessels.

The examiner has access to fine-tune the Doppler settings, such as the pulse repetition frequency (PRF) knob. To visualize small vessels with increased flow in the inflamed tissue, the PRF needs to be turned down to be able to pick up vascularity. If the PRF is set too high, very little presence of increased or even normal vascularity may be seen.

In this case, very little flow is seen within the entire ASC/perianal Doppler Color Power box. This is likely because of which incorrect use of instrumentation?

a. Overall gain is set too high
b. Overall gain is set too low
c. PRF is set too high
d. PRF is set too low

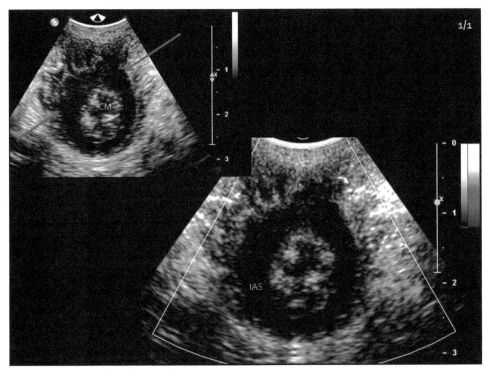

Fig. 42

CASE 20, FIGURES 43 AND 44

4. Figs. 43 and 44 demonstrate a right paraovarian lesion in a 36-year-old patient with chronic right lower quadrant pain. It measures $4.3 \times 3.7 \times 3.8$ cm with a volume of 32 mL (cm^3) and is unchanged from a previous exam 6 weeks ago. Answer the following:

   a. Is the contour of the lesion smooth or irregular? _____

   b. With normal machine settings, sound traveling through assumed similar tissue will automatically have the gain increased by the ultrasound system as it progresses from superficial to deep tissue in order to make like tissue appear the same superficially as well as deeply. This process is called "time gain compensation" (TGC). Sometimes this is referred to as "depth gain compensation." In other words, the gain will be increased in deeper tissue to compensate for the predictable absorption of sound. The examiner can additionally fine-tune the increased gain at the machine's TGC pod levels along the side of the control panel that approximate depth through the tissue. Absorption of the propagating sound is bound to occur; therefore, with the machine TGC preset, a patient's liver, for example, looks the same superficially as it does deeply. Does the overall echo pattern of the mass appear the same superficially as it does deeply? _____

   c. When tissue is abnormal, however, the automatic process of TGC will still occur.

   In diagnostic imaging, the examiner can take advantage of the presence of increased or decreased echoes beyond a structure. In fact, diagnostic criteria can include whether there is enhancement or shadowing beyond a structure. For example, a cyst will not absorb the sound because it is filled with fluid, so there will be increased echoes beyond the mass. Contrarily, a dense solid mass will absorb the sound, so there will be an acoustic shadow beyond the mass. The use of this nomenclature should be part of the exam reporting. Find the TGC pods on your ultrasound system and note that you can increase or decrease the gain at any level when you slide the pods to the right or to the left.

   In Fig. 43, note that the tissue beyond the lesion that is opposite from the transducer location appears increased in echogenicity (hyperechoic; see between the gold lines). Is this echo pattern increased ("posterior acoustic enhancement") or decreased ("posterior acoustic shadowing")? _____

5. The term "homogeneity" globally implies a consistent smooth echo pattern throughout a structure, whereas the term "heterogeneity" implies diffuse complexity of echoes. Focusing back to the lesion (Fig. 43), which of the following best describes it?

   a. It is heterogeneous, with multiple septae noted within and along the inner inferior peripheral luminal wall.

   b. It is homogeneous, with thick mural nodules noted at the inner inferior luminal wall.

   c. It is heterogeneous, with diffuse thin septations noted within the entire lesion.

   d. It is homogeneous, with diffuse low-level central echoes noted.

6. "Heterogeneity" can be further described. Is the echo pattern of the lesion "complex primarily cystic in appearance" or "complex primarily solid in appearance?" _____

7. Fig. 44. Doppler Color Power vascularity demonstrates all the following *except* which one?
   a. No flow within the septa
   b. Diffuse intralesional vascularity
   c. Peripheral flow at the luminal wall
   d. Increased flow adjacent to the lesion

8. If this were a first-time examination, conservative follow-up may demonstrate a resolved finding on a subsequent exam performed, for example, 2 months later. Although most ovarian lesions are temporary (functional and benign) and resolve in 4–6 weeks, this finding is unchanged since her exam conducted 6 weeks ago and carries an increased index of suspicion for pathology.

The exam was repeated in 8 weeks and was found to be of very similar appearance, with the same echo pattern. The size and contour remained the same. Sonographic findings are most consistent with:
   a. Endometrioma
   b. Hemorrhagic corpus luteum
   c. Paraovarian simple cyst
   d. Dermoid

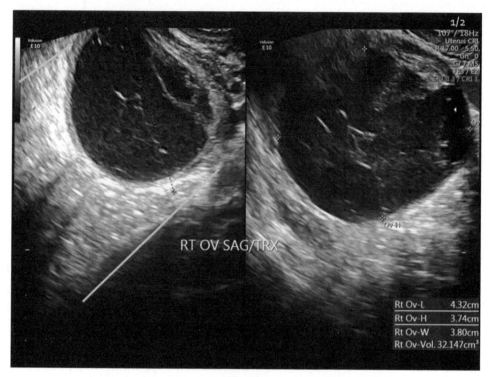

Fig. 43

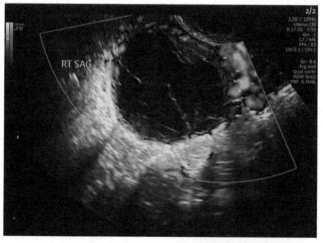

Fig. 44

CASE 21, FIGURE 45-48

9. Figs. 45–48 demonstrate transperineal 3D images of the pelvic floor in a 35-year-old patient with a sense of pelvic fullness and constipation. Fig. 45 is a 3D volume set of the pelvic floor using a 6–12 MHz EV transducer placed at the perineum with a depth of view at 5.5 cm, as indicated by the calipers alongside the A plane image. The 3D sweep angle was set at 75 degrees. The 3D volume set center reference point (CRP) in Fig. 45 is placed at the posterior aspect of the mid-urethra on the A plane and is seen at that same location on all three orthogonal planes. The colored dots are very small on these images; so, take advantage of the vertical (light blue) and horizontal (red) arrows on the screen that show the intersecting lines at the CRP. Identify the following labeled structures on the A sagittal plane:
   a. _____
   b. _____
   c. _____
   d. _____

10. Notice that the bowel is dilated proximal to the distal anal sphincter complex (ASC; Fig. 45, yellow arrows). In Fig. 46, the CRP has been moved by the examiner to which of the following locations (seen on all three planes of the 3D volume set indicated by the gold arrows)?
   a. Distal urethra/ASC interface
   b. Anterior vaginal wall/ASC interface
   c. Distal vaginal wall/ASC interface
   d. Proximal urethra/vaginal apex

11. In Fig. 46, compared with the echogenicity of the vagina, what is the echo pattern of the structure on which the CRP is located?
   a. Hypoechoic
   b. Isoechoic
   c. Hyperechoic

12. What are the approximate dimensions of the central irregular hypoechoic distal ASC mass (gold arrows in Fig. 46 and labeled "A" in Fig. 47)? (Measure in the Fig. 46 volume set using the caliper markings along the side. The large-to-large horizontal lines are 5 cm. The large-to-small horizontal lines are 1 cm, and the horizontal line-to-dot is 0.5 cm.) _____

13. The C plane in Fig. 46 is enlarged and rotated upright on the Z-axis for Fig. 47 to more intuitively visualize the pelvic floor complex in a transverse (axial) cut. The examiner should assess if the puboviseralis muscle (PVM) complex appears symmetric. Although the 3D sweep could have been set wider and angled more steeply through the volume to obtain the symphysis pubis and anterior lateral aspect of the PVM complex, it can be stated that the PVM complex is asymmetric and markedly irregular.
   a. On which side is there evidence of pelvic floor avulsion—left, right, or both? _____
   b. What does the structure labeled "A" (Fig. 47) most likely represent? _____
   c. What side does the structure labeled "B" (Fig. 47) represent? _____

14. Fig. 48 demonstrates two applications of the 3D rendered view of the pelvic floor complex, a live tissue option (screen left image) and a chroma option (screen right image).

   Subjectively, post-processed images may visualize the avulsion better. What the examiner sees is in the eyes of the beholder. The 3D capabilities available on your system are varied but can make a difference in your confidence about exam findings. There is a definite learning curve to acquire and master some of the 3D tool options; however, multiple visits from your vendor application specialist can help to learn and maximize the details. If you are not the one performing the exam, learn enough to make suggestions to your sonographer to maximize the ultrasound system options. Which image do you think demonstrates the anatomy more clearly? _____

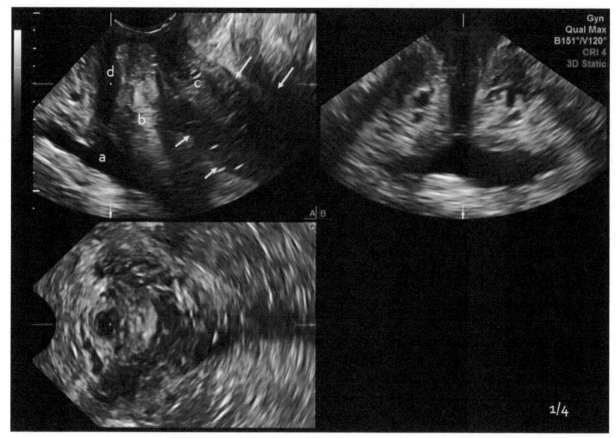

Fig. 45

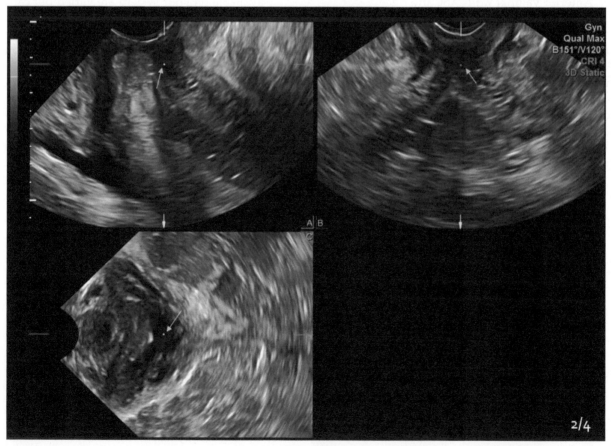

Fig. 46

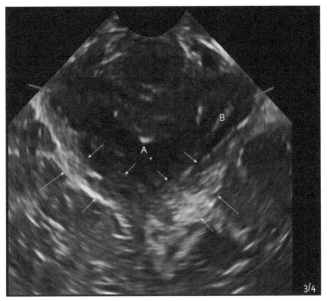

Fig. 47

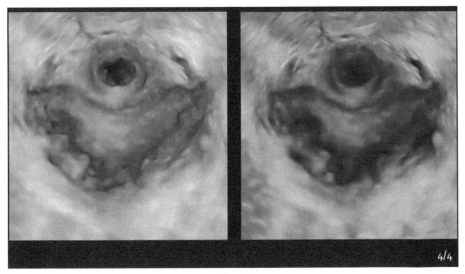

Fig. 48

CASE 22, FIGURES 49 AND 50

15. Figs. 49 and 50 are sagittal and transverse EV images of a normal uterus. With EV imaging using a 4–8 MHz transducer, the outer basal layer remains consistently thin throughout the cycle and is hyperechoic in echo pattern. It is the functional layer that thickens, changes in echo pattern as the cycle progresses, and sloughs off with menses. With the glandular changes and increase in density of the functional layer, the echo pattern goes from hypoechoic relative to the basal layer in the proliferative phase to isoechoic relative to the basal layer in the secretory phase.

The central cavity appears hyperechoic due to the meeting of the two apposing sides of the cavity wall. Therefore, during the proliferative phase, there is a clear delineation of the layers even as it thickens, creating a trilaminar appearance from the basal–functional–central cavity–functional–basal differentiation. The endometrial thickness is measured from the outer basal layer to the opposite outer basal layer.

Identify the labeled structures:

a. _____

b. _____

c. _____

d. _____

16. Fig. 50 is a transverse cut at the mid-uterus. Which segment of the *uterus* is labeled "e?" _____
   a. Subserosal
   b. Intramural
   c. Submucosal

17. Fig. 50. Which segment of the uterus is labeled "f?" _____
   a. Subserosal
   b. Intramural
   c. Submucosal

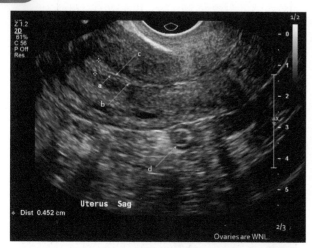

Fig. 49

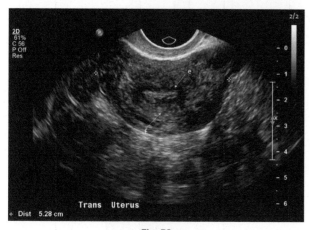

Fig. 50

CASE 23, FIGURES 51 AND 52

18. Figs. 51 and 52 are EV uterus images, using a 5–9 MHz EV transducer, of a 42-year-old multigravida presenting with menorrhagia or abnormal uterine bleeding, chronic pelvic pain that she describes as "aching in the middle of her uterus," and dyspareunia. The ovaries appear within normal limits bilaterally and are not presented here.
    a. In what position is the uterus? _____
    b. Is the overall echo pattern of the uterus homogeneous or heterogeneous? _____
19. As in all gynecologic ultrasound exams, when assessing patients with chronic pelvic pain, the exam should always include careful evaluation of the endometrium. The report should reflect the phase of the cycle related to the sonographic findings. The term "endometrial stripe" is never acceptable in describing the endometrium and should be removed from the GYN reporting vocabulary.

Note that there is very poor endometrial–myometrial differentiation present in Figs. 51 and 52. A definitive endometrium is not clear. The presence of pathology, however, may obscure normal anatomical identification. Though poorly seen, the endometrium area is diffusely increased in echogenicity compared with the myometrium, suggesting that the patient is in the secretory phase. Post-processing techniques can be employed to remove the mid-level to emphasize high versus low echoes.

Which of the following best describes the structures identified by arrows in Figs. 51 and 52?
    a. Multiple small hypoechoic endometrial lesions are noted along the endometrial–myometrial border, ranging in size from 1 to 5 mm in anteroposterior (AP) diameter.
    b. Diffuse small hypoechoic endometrial lesions are noted along the central endometrium, ranging in size from 1 to 5 mm in AP diameter.
    c. Diffuse small hyperechoic endometrial lesions are noted along the endometrial–myometrial border, ranging in size from 2 to 10 mm in AP diameter.
    d. Multiple small hypoechoic lesions are noted within the myometrium, ranging in size from 2 to 10 mm in AP diameter.
20. Which pattern of Doppler Color Power flow in Fig. 52 is demonstrated in this case (yellow arrows)?
    a. A paucity of flow within the area of interest
    b. An increase of flow within the area of interest
    c. Normal flow within the area of interest
    d. A peripheral flow pattern around an adjacent myometrial lesion
21. Findings are consistent with:
    a. Leiomyomata
    b. Uterine sarcoma
    c. Adenomyosis
    d. Endometrial carcinoma
    e. Concomitant adenomyosis and leiomyomata

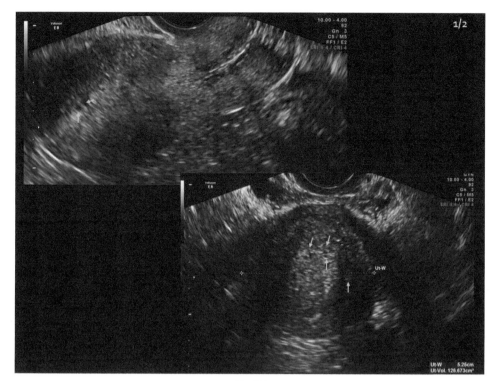

Fig. 51

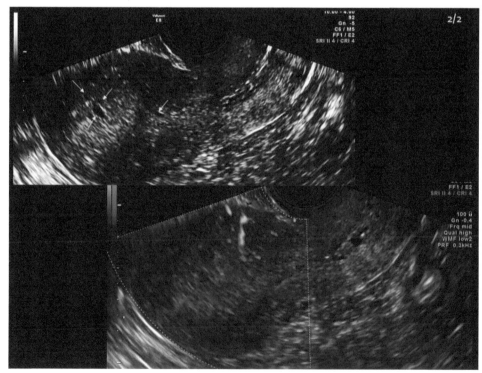

Fig. 52

CASE 24, FIGURES 53 AND 54

22. Figs. 53 and 54 demonstrate an abnormal hetero-geneous transverse cut at the mid-uterus, using a 4–8 MHz EV transducer, in a 27-year-old nullipa-rous woman with menorrhagia. The entire area is comprised of a large intrauterine lesion. What is the uterine width? Use calipers along the side of the image to measure. _____
    a. What is the typical uterine width? _____
    b. In your report, describe the lesion in terms of:
        i. Location. Is it myomatous, endometrial, left side, right side, anterior, or posterior? _____
        ii. Contour. Is it smooth, jagged, irregular, thin walled, or thick walled? _____
        iii. Shape. Is it oblong, bilobular, trapezoidal, oval, or serpigenous? _____
        iv. Echo pattern. Is it anechoic, hypoechoic, hyperechoic, complex primarily cystic in appearance, or complex primarily solid in appearance? _____
23. In Fig. 54, the thin hyperechoic rim around the le-sion is indicated by the gold arrows. This is the displaced basal layer of the endometrium sur-rounding the lesion. The two linear red lines dem-onstrate where the endometrium is not seen be-cause of displacement of the uterine mass into the endometrial cavity that originated here. The free fluid (indicated by ff) surrounding the lesion within the endometrial cavity is presumably pres-ent as a function of bleeding. Which of the follow-ing is the most likely diagnosis?
    a. Multiple endometrial polyps
    b. Submucosal leiomyomata
    c. Intramural leiomyomata
    d. Endometrial hemorrhage

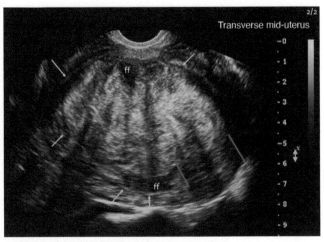

Fig. 54

CASE 25, FIGURE 55

24. Fig. 55 includes a transperineal 3D volume set of the pelvic floor. The acquisition A plane is sagittal, the B plane is transverse, and the C plane is a coro-nal view. The irregular anechoic triangularly/oval shaped structure seen on all three planes is well visualized because the center reference point (CRP) has been moved from the original middle of the sweep location through the volume to bring that point of interest onto all three orthogonal planes. Note that the location of the CRP is *not* at midline and that the only orthogonal plane includ-ing visualization of the urethra is the C plane. This improves the relative anatomy of this abnormal pelvic floor. The C plane was then pulled out of the volume set and rotated on the Z-axis to bring the anatomy into a more logical upright position (screen bottom right).
    From what structure does this anechoic mass appear to originate?
    a. Posterior urethra
    b. Anterior vagina
    c. Posterior vagina
    d. Central vagina
    e. Anterior rectum
    f. Posterior rectum
25. In what direction is the lesion protruding? (Fig. 55)
    a. Anteriorly
    b. Posteriorly
    c. Right
    d. Left
26. Note that the lesion volume is calculated by measuring the three planes of the lesion. If you or

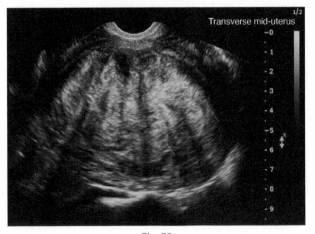

Fig. 53

your sonographer did not measure the lesion during the exam, but you need the dimensions now, you can calculate the volume post exam. Using the calipers along the side of the image, re-measure the lesion. Are the measurements the same? _____

27. Some would simplify the sonographic diagnosis as a vaginal cyst. Which *two* of the following

would *not* be in your differential diagnosis for this appearance?
  a. Rectal abscess
  b. Bartholin's duct cyst
  c. Epidermal inclusion cyst
  d. Mullerian cyst
  e. Urethral diverticulum

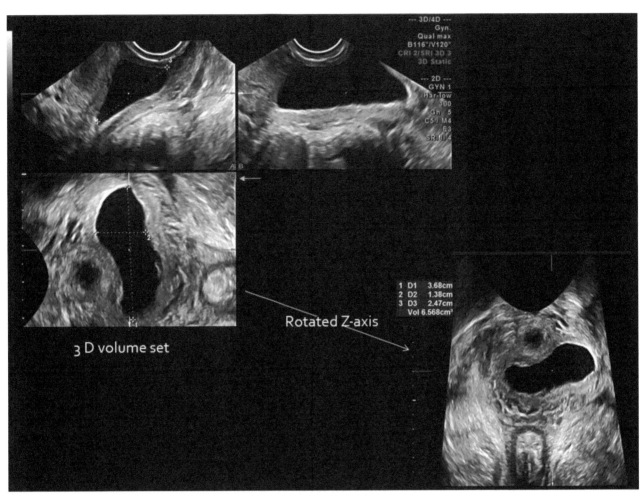

Fig. 55

CASE 26, FIGURES 56–61

28. Figs. 56–61 are images of a 49-year-old woman who presented to her provider with increasing lower abdominal pain. She is status post (s/p) total vaginal hysterectomy (TVH). Her left ovary was well visualized and appeared within normal limits, and is not shown here. Gold arrows point to the calipers in Figs. 56 and 57. The following questions are based on the right adnexal images. The typical normal ovary measures $1 \times 2 \times 3$ cm, although a normally functioning ovary will have modest increase in volume throughout the cycle with the formation and resolution of follicles and a corpus luteum. Using the prolate ellipsoid formula ($L \times H \times W \times 0.52$), the normal volume is 3.12 mL (cm^3).

What is the ovarian volume in this case? _____

29. In Figs. 56–58, the right ovary is comprised of a complex mass. Describe the mass in terms of:
  a. Contour. Is it smooth, jagged, irregular, thin walled, or thick walled? _____
  b. Shape. Is it oblong, bilobular, trapezoidal, oval, or serpigenous? _____
  c. Echo pattern. Is it anechoic, hypoechoic, hyperechoic, homogeneous, or heterogeneous? _____

30. Figs. 59 and 60 focus on the oblong irregular hyperechoic subcomponent of the mass seen at the superior aspect of the mass (bottom of the screen). Applying Doppler Color Power to the mass to obtain information about the vascular patterns of the mass is important. Merely turning on Doppler Color Flow may elicit little or increased flow. If there appears to be very little flow, remember that preprogrammed ultrasound system settings will

often demonstrate poor vascular pickup, when, in actuality, even normal vessels have an abundance of flow within the normal tissue at the right setting; therefore, the examiner should turn down the pulse repetition frequency (PRF) knob to where the vessels begin to blush and then go back up a step or two to where the real flow level is depicted, as is seen here. This cannot be done as a post-processing tool at a workstation.

Fig. 59 demonstrates multiple ill-patterned vessels within the solid appearing subcomponent of the lesion, as well as within vertical septae seen extending into the mass on the 2D image. The multiplicity of vessels is increasingly concerning when the 3D rendered image is seen in Fig. 60. Is the Doppler Color Power visible within and/or around the mass subcomponent? _____

31. With the abundance of Doppler Color vascularity, a Doppler Spectral Waveform is extremely important to add to the assessment. Interpreting the significance of individual vessel velocity values is complicated. Given the infinite variability of normal as well as abnormal vessel velocity ranges, actual calculated velocity of a single vessel would be impossible to comparatively assess. What has been found to be consistent is the ratio of various vessel velocity relationships during systole and diastole.

The typical resistive index (RI) of the normal ovary is greater than 0.4, which is obtained by subtracting the end-diastolic velocity (EDV) from the peak systolic velocity (PSV), which is then divided by the PSV. This index is calculated by the ultrasound system when the spectral waveform is measured but can be calculated post exam by measuring systolic and diastolic values on the image. Some use the pulsatility index (PI) that is calculated by subtracting EDV from PSV, which is then divided by the *mean* diastolic velocity. Normal PI is thought to be greater than 1.0. This cannot be calculated post exam because the mean velocity must be measured on the waveform.

How abnormal vascular flow changes from normal flow alters those ratios. With neoangiogenesis of fast forming vessels, such as in a malignant lesion, the elastic middle (muscular layer) part of the vessel layers is thought to fail to form quickly enough to retain normal vessel wall recoil during diastole and systole. Consequently, the diastolic flow increases and the normal resistance to blood flow decreases, thereby causing the indices to decrease. Additionally, aberrant ill-patterned vessels form within the lesion.

Fig. 61 demonstrates the Doppler velocities throughout the cardiac cycle and the spectral waveform indices (upper right-hand corner). What is the RI for this ovary? _____

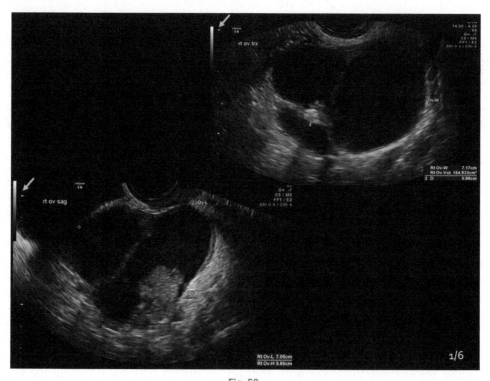

Fig. 56

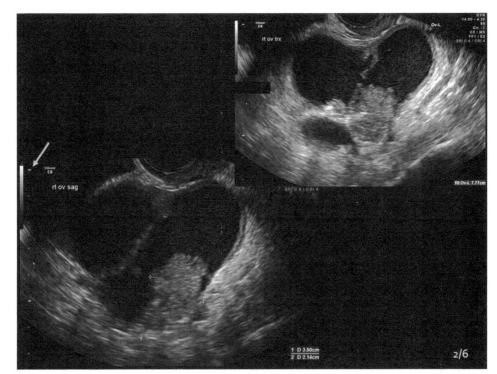

Fig. 57

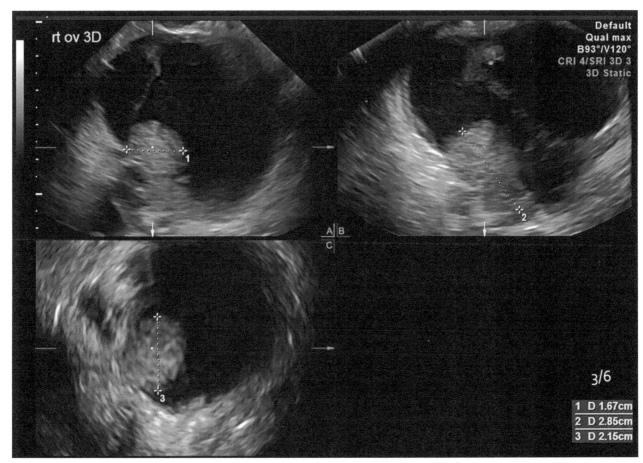

Fig. 58

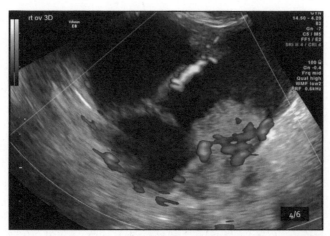

Fig. 59

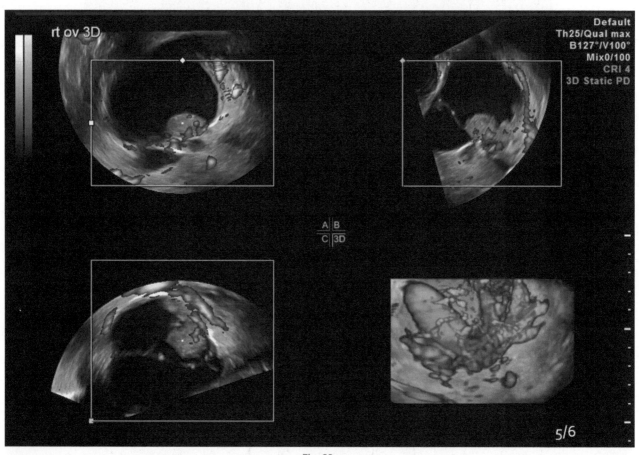

Fig. 60

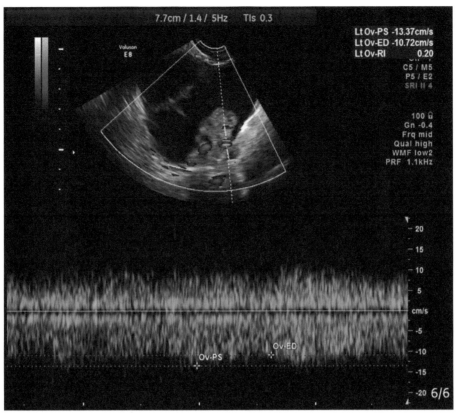

Fig. 61

CASE 27, FIGURES 62–65

32. Figs. 62–65 are images, using a 5–9 MHz EV transducer, of a 21-year-old s/p fourth-degree tear at delivery and postpartum repair who presented 4 days later with searing perineal pain. The 2D EV transducer is placed perpendicular to the table at the posterior vaginal wall directly above the anal sphincter complex (ASC) and can be scanned in both the sagittal as well as transverse planes by rotating 90 degrees.

    a. Fig. 62 is a transperineal exam of the ASC at what level? _____

    The structures labeled "A" and "B" are the indicators of the level.

    b. Which side of the patient is structure "B"? _____

    c. From where to where (as if on a clock) is the internal anal sphincter (IAS) disrupted? _____

33. The patient barely tolerated placement of the transducer at the perineum, so the transducer was placed with a very light touch over increased gel at the posterior vaginal wall. In addition to describing the evident IAS disruption, note the abnormal perianal tissue above the disruption and under the transducer at the posterior vaginal wall, as seen in Figs. 63 and 64. Note that the calipers in Fig. 63 show that the ASC is not even seen with the marked perianal thickening measuring more than 4 cm in depth.

This area appears heterogeneous with poor distinction of tissue margins that are difficult to distinguish. Additionally, some of this area appears isoechoic to the surrounding tissue. The examiner can post-process the image to knock out mid-level echoes and improve border delineation as in the bottom left image of Fig. 63. Note the presence of diffuse punctate echogenic foci within the perianal tissue (gold arrows in the bottom left image of Fig. 63). This likely represents the presence of air within the tissue.

In the top image, this area is measured. What are the dimensions? _____

34. Fig. 64 demonstrates the surrounding perianal soft tissue without and with Color Power Doppler. Notice that the central area demonstrates increased vascularity. Does the Color Power overlie a more or less dense area of perianal tissue on the 2D gray scale image? _____

35. Compare top and bottom images of Fig. 65. The top is a 2D Color Power Doppler image and the bottom is a 3D rendered image of the vascularity. One can appreciate the difference in seeing one slice of increased vascularity (top) and the volume of increased vascularity in the 3D image (bottom).

When 2D imaging suggests increased flow, the 3D rendered image (Fig. 65) often brings surprisingly enhanced appreciation of additive increased flow to a hypervascularized area. Write a detailed description of your findings.

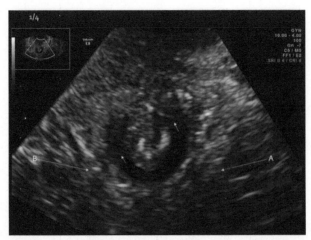

Fig. 62

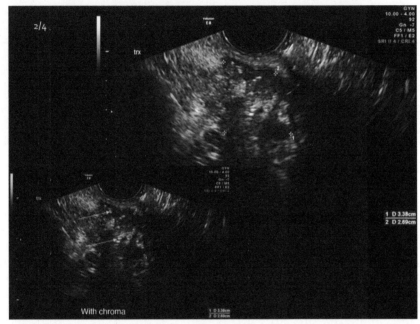

Fig. 63

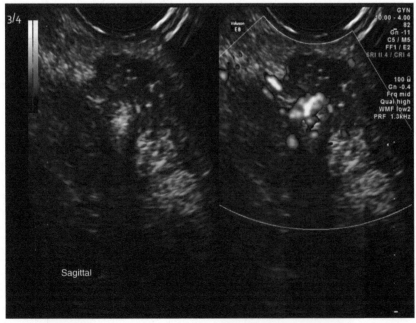

Fig. 64

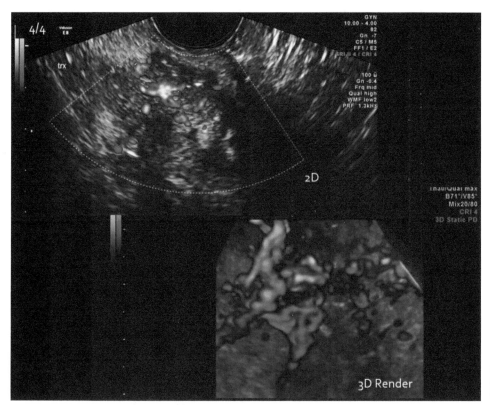

Fig. 65

CASE 28, FIGURES 66–68

36. Figs. 66–68 are two images pulled out of a 3D volume set (red asterisk in Fig. 66 indicates A and B planes) of the uterus using a 5–9 MHz curvilinear EV transducer to assess the location of an intrauterine device (IUD) in a patient experiencing midline pelvic pain since IUD placement. The uterus is anteverted and retroflexed (Fig. 66) with the fundus poorly seen because it is retroflexed (white arrows) and partially out of the full field of view.

   Appreciate that if only 2D is performed, the IUD location may erroneously be perceived to be in correct location because the coronal C plane cannot be obtained on a 2D exam.

   The two orthogonal A and B planes shown in Fig. 66 are which of the following cuts?
   a. Transverse and sagittal
   b. Sagittal and transverse
   c. Transverse and coronal
   d. Sagittal and coronal

37. When a 3D volume set is made, there will be a center reference point (CRP) dot, "X", or cross (depending on the machine vendor) at the middle of the initial volume on all planes of the initial images. In Fig. 66, the CRP is not placed on the uterus (green arrows). The CRP is where the initial 3D sweep would place it, which is at the center of the volume. With any volume set, the CRP should be moved to the area of interest by the examiner. In this case, it should be moved to the IUD on either image which will centralize the same area of interest on the other orthogonal planes as well. The anatomy posterior to the uterus in this image is insignificant and unnecessary to demonstrate.

   Note that the CRP is moved to the IUD in Figs. 67 and 68.

   See the gold arrow in Fig. 67. Is the stem of the IUD located centrally within the C plane view of the endometrial canal? Yes or No _____

38. When 3D imaging is used, as in Fig. 68 where the C plane is pulled out from the volume set, the examiner has multiple tools available to improve visualization at areas of interest in order to visualize the arms. The use of chroma options may help to accentuate borders of the IUD (right upper image) and bring the arms into better view.

   Notice that the CRP was moved to just right of the stem in Fig. 68 (green arrow); however, it could have been moved ONTO the arm which would result in the volume set demonstrating both the arms and stem in one image.

   See gold arrows in Fig. 68. Are the arms of the IUD located centrally with the endometrial canal? Yes or No _____

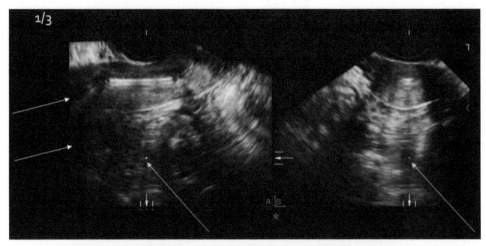

Fig. 66

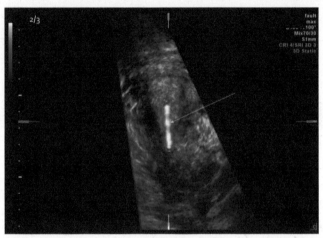

Fig. 67

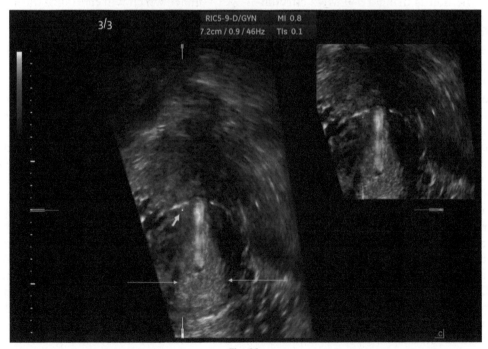

Fig. 68

CASE 29, FIGURES 69-71

39. Figs. 69–71 demonstrate three distinct planes of the internal anal sphincter/external anal sphincter (IAS/EAS) complex in the same patient using a transperineal 5–9 MHz EV transducer. At what level is Fig. 69 transverse image taken? _____

40. Identify labeled structures of Fig. 69:
    a. Label A _____
    b. Label B _____
    c. Label C _____

41. Fig. 70 demonstrates the anal sphincter complex (ASC) at the distal IAS level, where the peripheral hyperechoic symmetric intact EAS is well visualized surrounding the IAS. This is a 2D image that could have better equalized the lateral aspects of the EAS by slight rotation of the EV transducer; nevertheless, the EAS is clearly intact.

    Identify which labeled side is the left and which is the patient's right side.
    a. Label E _____
    b. Label F _____

42. Fig. 71 is a rotated C plane of a transperineal pelvic floor 3D volume set using a 5–9 MHz EV transducer. Note the "C" letter on the bottom right of the image, indicating that this image is the C plane pulled out of a 3D volume set (gold arrow). One can tell that the center reference point was not moved anteriorly enough to include pubic symphysis on the original acquisition plane because the anterior pubic symphysis/pubovisceralis muscle (PVM) complex attachment is not seen on the C plane (red). The volume set sweep was wide enough to visualize the lateral aspect of the PVM complex. Can the examiner comment on the presence or absence of an avulsion from this image? _____

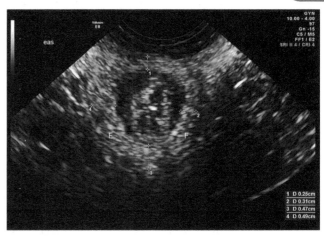

Fig. 70

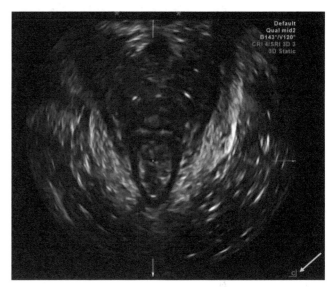

Fig. 71

CASE 30, FIGURE 72

43. Fig. 72 is an image from an EV exam, using a 4–8 MHz EV transducer, of a small hemorrhagic clot formed following an endometrial biopsy procedure performed just prior to the ultrasound exam. It demonstrates 2D sagittal and transverse cuts of the (same) clot at the lower uterine segment endometrial cavity. Think about directions in the patient when using an EV transducer and why the same clot looks different in the two planes. Explain the difference in appearances *as related to the plane and the body*. _____

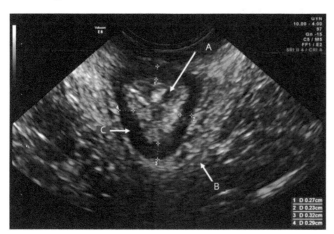

Fig. 69

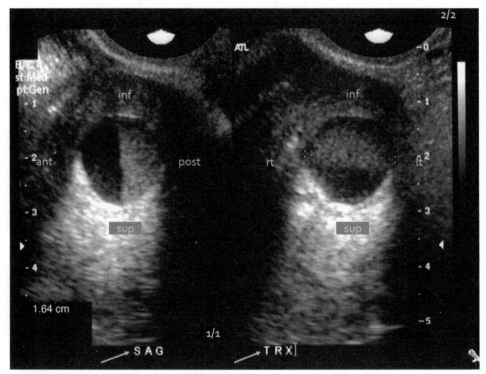

Fig. 72

CASE 31, FIGURE 73

44. Fig. 73. Sometimes ovaries are hard to visualize, especially when there is pathology. The left ovary appeared within normal limits in both exams and is not presented here. Fig. 73 demonstrates the right ovary of a 40-year-old patient using a 4–8 MHz EV transducer. Her last menstrual period was 1 week ago. A previous exam 8 weeks ago demonstrated an abnormal echo pattern of the right ovary at an outside institution.
   a. The subcomponent lesion within the ovary is being measured in the image. See yellow arrows. Does the ovary measure normal in size? _____

   b. Is the contour of the ovary smooth or irregular? _____

   c. Are normal follicles visualized? _____

45. Which of the following best describes the echo pattern of the ovary?
   a. Heterogeneous with an irregular hyperechoic subcomponent
   b. Central homogeneous echo pattern
   c. Complex primarily cystic appearance
   d. Homogeneous solid appearance
   e. Heterogeneous with an irregular hypoechoic peripheral mass
46. There is no evidence of vascular flow of this ovary as seen on the top Doppler Color Power image. Because no flow is seen, was the pulse repetition frequency likely set too low or too high? _____
47. Based on the 2D imaging, which of the following is the most likely diagnosis?
   a. Simple follicular cyst
   b. Hemorrhagic corpus luteum
   c. Dermoid
   d. Borderline mucinous tumor

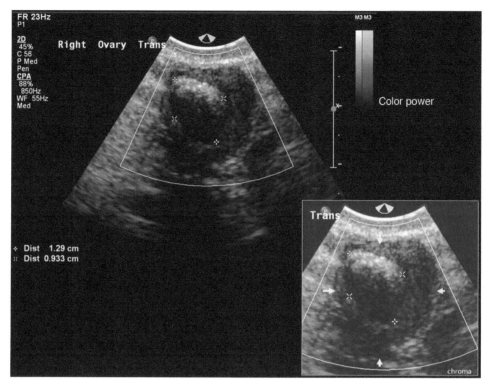

Fig. 73

CASE 32, FIGURE 74

48. Fig. 74. The normal female urethra measures 4 cm in length, and the neck is typically 6 mm in an anteroposterior (AP) diameter. Fig. 74 demonstrates a transperineal midline sagittal cut of the urethra at rest using a 5–9 MHz EV transducer. The length of this urethra is 3.4 cm, and the AP diameter of the neck is 7.1 mm.

The entire urethra is not visualized. What could account for this discrepancy? _____

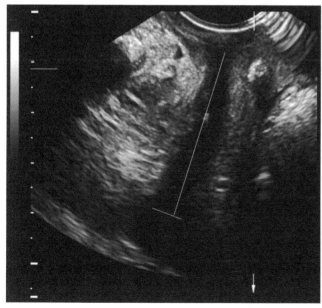

Fig. 74

CASE 33, FIGURES 75 AND 76

49. Fig. 75 is a transperineal transverse bladder image of the same patient with the EV transducer placed halfway into the vagina. The bladder is partially filled. The gold arrow points to an irregular oblong structure within the bladder that appears like a free-floating mass in this plane.

The transducer is rotated 90 degrees along the red line in the suspicious area as seen in Fig. 76. It now appears to be contiguous with the bladder wall, not a separate mass, urine imaged on both sides of the slice. This is an example of how important assessing anatomy in two planes is, especially in the presence of what may be perceived to be an abnormality that appears very real in one plane.

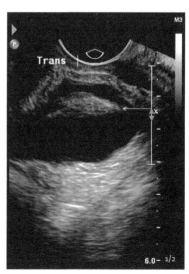

Fig. 75

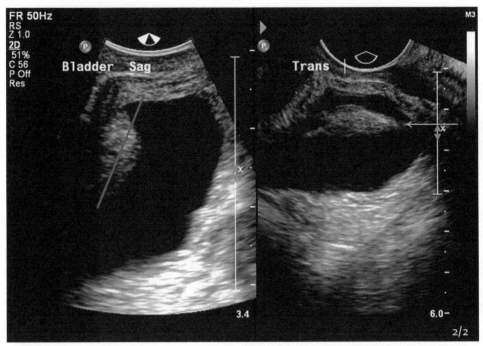

Fig. 76

CASE 34, FIGURES 77 AND 78

50. Fig. 77 is a midline sagittal image of an anteverted uterus, using a 5–9 MHz EV transducer, in a patient with a history of abnormal uterine bleeding. The patient states this is day 6 of her cycle, although she says it is hard to tell sometimes as she is nearly always bleeding.

    Answer the following:

    a. Are the functional and basal layers indistinctly or distinctly visualized? _____

    b. Is the normal basal layer seen at the endometrial center or at the endometrial periphery? _____

    c. What is the normal maximum endometrial thickness during the secretory phase? _____

    d. Using the calipers along the side of the image, what does this endometrial thickness measure? _____

51. Fig. 78 demonstrates Color Power Doppler of a 3D volume set on the same patient from an initial transverse sweep of the endometrium. Now the endometrium is seen as an intracavity mass with a focal area of vascularity. With careful evaluation of the cumulative three orthogonal planes and the rendered image, the vascular pattern can be appreciated. Does the vascular complex extend along the lateral left endometrial peripheral border or does it appear to extend centrally into the endometrium? _____

52. Each of the three orthogonal planes demonstrates one slice of the mass vascularity. The 3D rendered image demonstrates the cumulative appearance of a cluster of increased vessels that extend centrally into the bulky endometrial lesion. Of the following, which is the most likely diagnosis for this appearance?

    a. Late secretory phase of the endometrium
    b. Endometrial carcinoma
    c. Endometrial polyp
    d. Hemorrhagic clot
    e. Submucosal leiomyoma

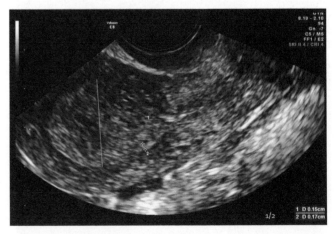

Fig. 77

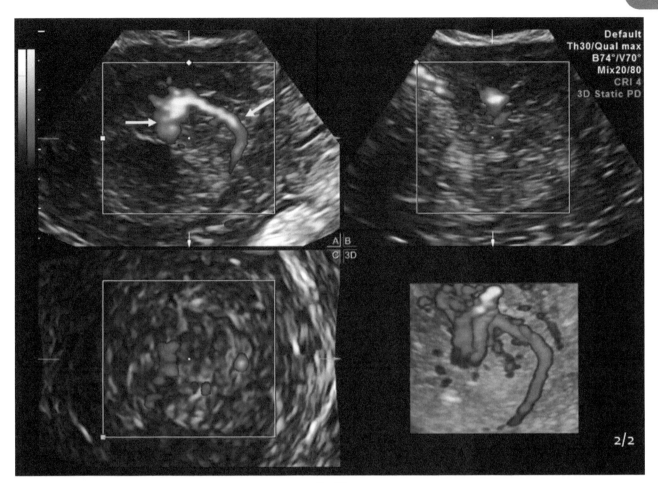

Fig. 78

CASE 35, FIGURE 79

53. Fig. 79 is a magnified transperineal sagittal image of the bladder using a 4–8 MHz EV transducer.

   a. Is the measured anteroposterior thickness of the bladder wall within normal limits? _____

   b. Images are often taken without calipers at the time of the exam. There may later be areas deemed as good, if not better, locations to obtain additional measurements. Using the calipers on the image, what is the gold arrow line thickness? _____

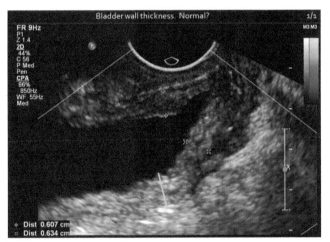

Fig. 79

Case Reviews 36–55

Outline

TOPIC 3, FIGURE 80

1. Fig. 80. Topic: Approach to Exam Assessment

   How does one assess an ultrasound examination in order to thoroughly interpret the findings and create the report? Always start with global descriptions and then progress to specific details. Check caliper scales, depth of image views, relative anatomy, and echo patterns. Obtain parameter measurements. When pathology is present, describe size, contour, and altered echo pattern. Include how pathology affects the absorption of sound with description of evidence of enhanced through transmission or posterior acoustic shadowing. Use Doppler to assess vascularization. Include Doppler spectral waveform indices when patterns are altered. Perform at least two resistive indices (RI) at hypervascularized area of interest.

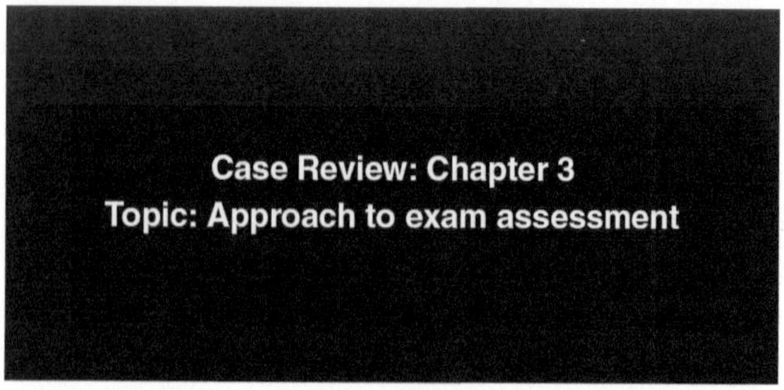

Case Review: Chapter 3
Topic: Approach to exam assessment

Fig. 80

CASE 36, FIGURES 81-83

2. Figs. 81 and 82 are schematic drawings of the midsagittal pelvis. Figs. 81 and 82 demonstrate anteverted (AV) and retroverted (RV) uterus positions, respectively, each without and with a full bladder. The blue arrows in both the figures represent the transducer location on the anterior abdominopelvic wall just above the symphysis to assess the transabdominal pelvic view relative to the uterus. The varied positions of the uterus, however, influence the effectiveness of image quality with this approach. To optimally image the uterus when performing a transabdominal exam, the transducer should be perpendicular to the anatomy of interest; therefore, the bladder must be filled to retrovert the uterus and orient the sound-absorbing small bowel superiorly.

   By filling the bladder, an acoustic "window" is created (Fig. 81, screen right) through which the sound travels with little absorption to visualize the uterus behind it. When the bladder is full, the position of the AV uterus is now RV enough that the transducer will be closer to perpendicular to the central endometrial lining which will improve the image resolution. Partially filling the bladder will enhance the image only minimally and pathology can be missed. Remember that three out of four women have an AV uterus making it the most common examiner experience. Either have the patient drink more water and wait to do the transabdominal exam or perform the endovaginal (EV) portion of the exam while the bladder is filling if you must still get the overall pelvis portion of the exam.

When the bladder is full, the RV uterus may not change in its position at all (Fig. 82, screen right). Steeply orienting the transducer to visualize the central endometrial lining perpendicularly will likely remain suboptimal. The examiner could move the abdominal transducer toward the patient's head and then angle caudally (gold arrows) to try to approach the endometrium perpendicularly through the full bladder, although with varying degrees of success; therefore, the RV uterus is often substandard in transabdominal imaging, regardless of how much more the bladder is filled.

3. Fig. 83 (A–D) demonstrates four examples of the midline sagittal image of the AV uterus.
   a. Which images are made with EV transducers? _____
   b. Is the bladder full enough to assess the entire uterus of image A? _____
   c. On which image of Fig. 83 is the cervical canal interface as well seen as the endometrial canal on the same image? _____
   d. Which images demonstrate the endometrium well enough to identify the phase of the endometrial cycle? _____

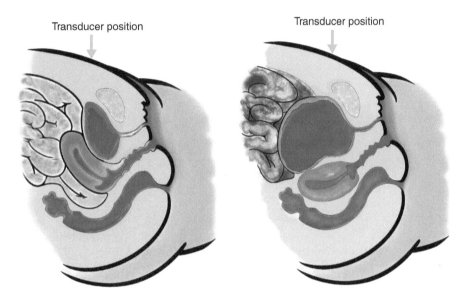

Fig. 81

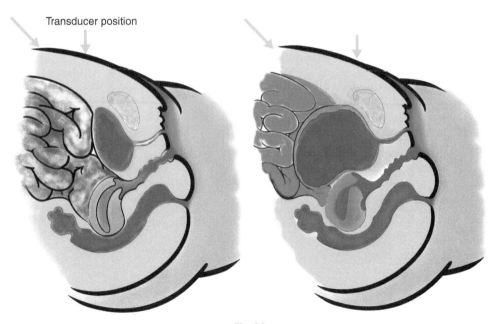

Fig. 82

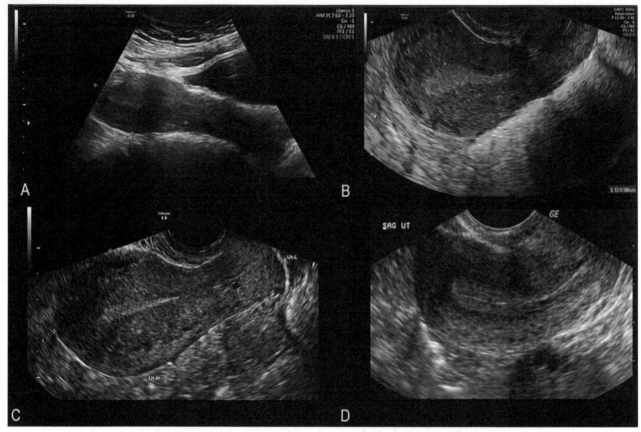

Fig. 83

CASE 37, FIGURES 84 AND 85

4. Fig. 84. Unfortunately, patients often feel discomfort when vaginal ultrasound examinations are performed. When the transducer is placed "straight" into the pelvic floor anatomy from the introitus (green line), it will bump against the uterus and bladder. Purposeful placement and angulation of the endovaginal (EV) transducer to align with the anatomy seen on the monitor is crucial to identify and assess predictable as well as altered pelvic anatomy.

Remember, the vagina extends posteriorly relative to the horizontal table on which the patient is lying, so the transducer needs to be angled down (towards the patient's back) as it is placed into the vaginal canal. **Watch the screen.** You can follow yourself towards the anatomy of interest. As related to the anatomy of Fig. 84, how would the transducer have to be moved to bring the following into view?
a. Uterine fundus _____
b. Bladder _____
c. Urethra _____
d. Rectum _____

5. Fig. 85 depicts EV images of a (A) RV uterus and (B) an AV uterus. Any view of anatomy can be strengthened by directing the sound towards it; for example, in what direction would the transducer have to be directed to better see *the lower uterine segment* for each image?
a. Image A _____
b. Image B _____
c. In what phase of the menstrual cycle is the uterus in image A? _____
d. In what phase of the menstrual cycle is the uterus in image B? _____

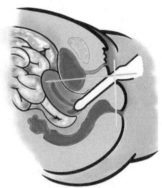

Be careful.
Introducing the transducer straight in (green line) would:
1. Demonstrate the posterior bladder.
2. Miss the vaginal apex– lower uterine segment interface.
3. Make the patient uncomfortable.

Fig. 84

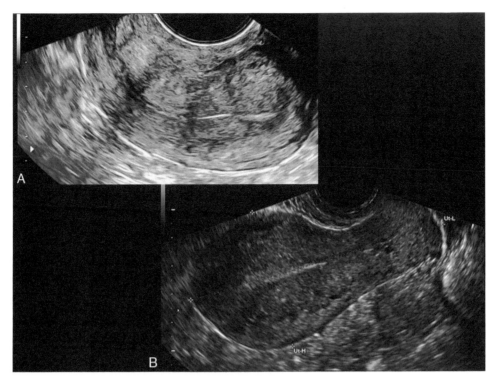

Fig. 85

CASE 38, FIGURE 86

6. Fig. 86 demonstrates a transperineal 3D volume set of the pelvic floor using a 5–9 MHz endovaginal transducer. The acquisition sweep is a sagittal A plane (screen top left). Remember, the B plane (screen top right) is perpendicular to the A plane along the red line and the C plane (screen bottom left) is coronal to the A plane along the blue line. The volume sweep angle is arbitrarily set at 75 degrees. The small faintly colored yellow, red, and blue center reference points are at the intersection of all three orthogonal planes (A, B, C) at which is located a complex lesion at the *posterior vaginal wall*. The rendered image is not shown.
   a. What does the lesion measure (calipers are at A and B planes)? _____
   b. How would you describe the measured lesion (best seen on B plane) in terms of shape—oval, trapezoidal, round, rectangular, or serpiginous? _____
   c. Is it hyperechoic, isoechoic, or hypoechoic relative to the distal anterior vagina (at red)? _____
7. How would you describe the measured lesion in terms of location relative to the urethra and bladder? (A plane; screen top left)
   a. Is it anterior or posterior to the mid-urethra? _____
   b. Is it anterior, posterior, inferior, or superior to the bladder? _____

8. As the A plane is sagittal *on the patient*, what are the B and C planes? _____
9. In which of the three orthogonal planes is the urethra *not* seen? _____
10. The screen bottom right image of Fig. 86 is the C plane rotated upright, which may seem more intuitive to see the anatomy. The rendered image is not present. Note that the green arrows demonstrate an additional round lesion along the right lateral vaginal wall that is well circumscribed, but hyperechoic to the vagina. It also demonstrates diffuse punctate echogenic foci; therefore, there are two vaginal lesions. Using the calipers along the side of the A plane, what does the second lesion measure? _____
11. Which of the following is your sonographic diagnosis of the two lesions?
    a. Urethral diverticulum
    b. Vaginal cyst
    c. Rectocele
    d. Vaginal myomata

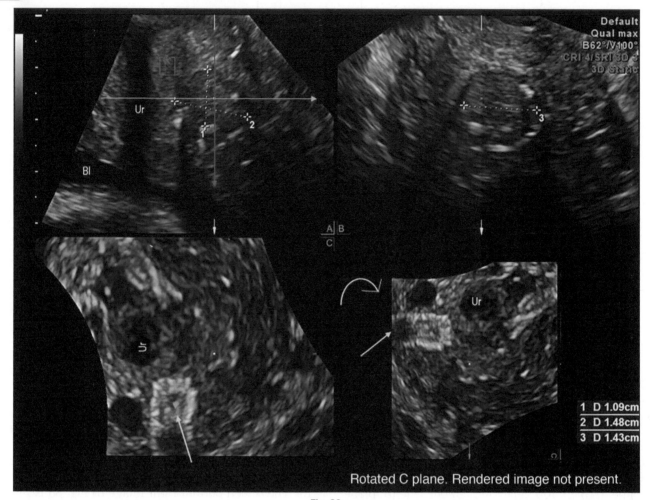

Fig. 86

CASE 39, FIGURES 87 AND 88

12. Fig. 87 is a 2D transperineal image using a 5–9 MHz transducer placed halfway into the vagina and angled slightly anteriorly to view the nearly empty bladder of a 58-year-old woman with urinary incontinence.

    Which of the following would best describe the bladder wall?
    a. The wall is diffusely thickened and irregular.
    b. The wall is thickened and smooth.
    c. The wall is irregular and of normal thickness.
    d. The wall is smooth and of normal thickness.

13. Fig. 88 is a transperineal 3D volume set of the bladder (same patient), including the 3D rendered image (screen bottom right) using a 5–9 MHz endovaginal transducer. It is evident on all three planes that the bladder wall irregularity is diffuse. The center reference point has been brought to the irregular bladder wall. The examiner can improve the initial 3D rendered image by bringing down the (green) line of reference from the initial top of the screen into the area of interest which is at the partially filled bladder on A and B planes. Subsequently, the rendered image well depicts the bladder wall as diffusely trabeculated.

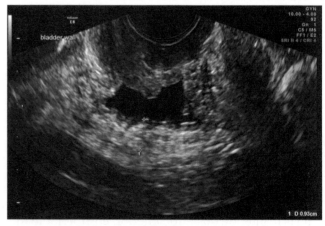

Fig. 87

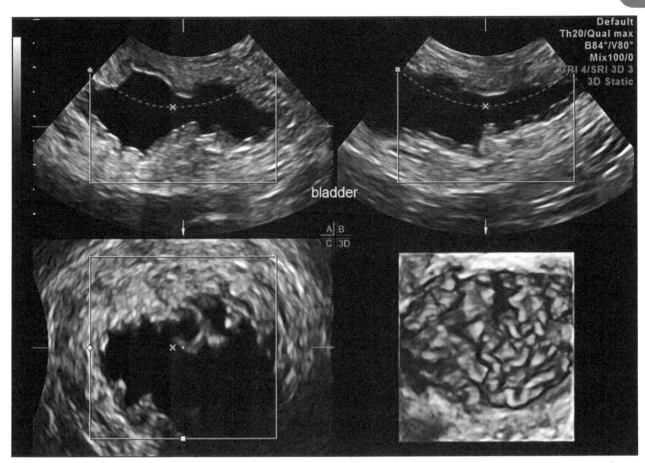

Fig. 88

CASE 40, FIGURE 89

Note that Fig. 89 (another patient) differs from the volume set of Fig. 90. The center reference point (CRP) of the volume set for Fig. 89 is seen in the center of the volume, which is the initial location once a sweep is done, not at the wall. In this case, it happens to be placed in the idle middle of what structure? _____

Additionally, the line of reference (LOR) remains higher than the concerning posterior luminal wall; therefore, the 3D rendered image (bottom right) appears more "far away" and less sharp. This is a subtle example of how bringing the CRP and LOR down *to* the anatomy of interest enhances the rendered image. The examiner can optimize the volume set by moving the CRP and LOR to the area of interest. This can also be done post exam at the ultrasound system or a workstation, but only if the volume is saved.

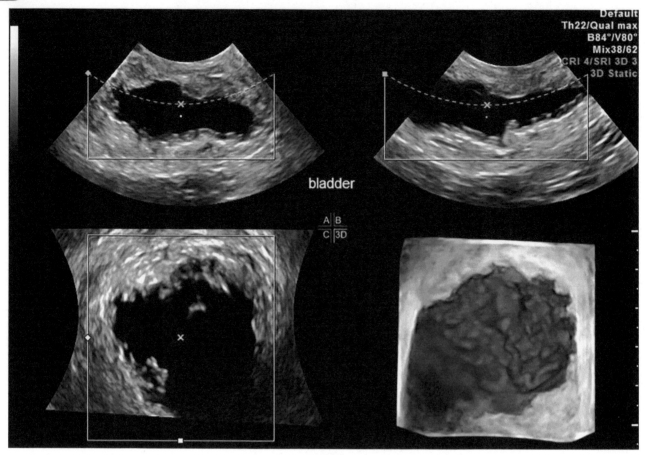

Fig. 89

CASE 41, FIGURES 90–93

14. A 24-year-old woman presented to her gynecologist after gradual swelling and, now, with severe pain in her right labium. Figs. 90–93 are images of the labia using a 5–9 MHz endovaginal transducer placed at each labium. Fig. 90 is of the normal left labium in sagittal and transverse planes. The measurement was taken for relative comparison with the swollen labium, which is seen in Fig. 92, where the calipers along the B plane right side can be used to measure on the screen.

a. What does the right labium measure? _____

b. Fig. 91 does not have the calipers along the side because the image is zoomed around the centered labium, removing the calipers; so, a post-exam measurement could not be taken on this image and instead could be measured on the 3D volume set of Fig. 92. The purpose of Fig. 92 is to demonstrate Color Power Doppler, which was initiated to assess vascular flow of the abnormal right side. Note that the pre-programmed initial Gyn pre-settings of Color Power Doppler create the appearance of practically no flow on the image.

Considering the amount of pain that the patient is experiencing, an error in the depiction of vascularity with a paucity of right labial Color Power Doppler should be considered with this appearance. Additionally, with the amount of unilateral swelling present, it is crucial to remember that the ultrasound system's pre-established pulse repetition frequency (PRF) Gyn pre-settings may be set too high. To demonstrate actual flow of this area, the PRF should be reduced. By reducing the PRF, Fig. 92 demonstrates a much more realistic rendering of the right labium's overall vascularity, especially of the 3D rendered image at the bottom right. Fig. 93 demonstrates the difference between the preset Color Power Doppler pickup and the correctly adjusted markedly increased flow.

Does the corrected Color Power Doppler vascular pattern appearance of the right labium suggest focal or diffuse hypervascularity? _____

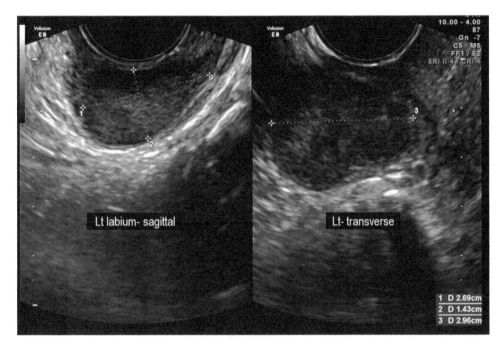

Fig. 90

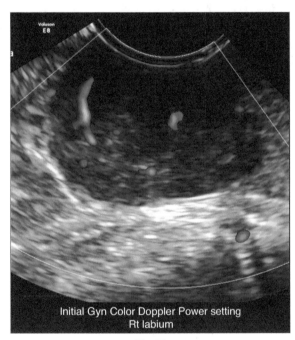

Fig. 91

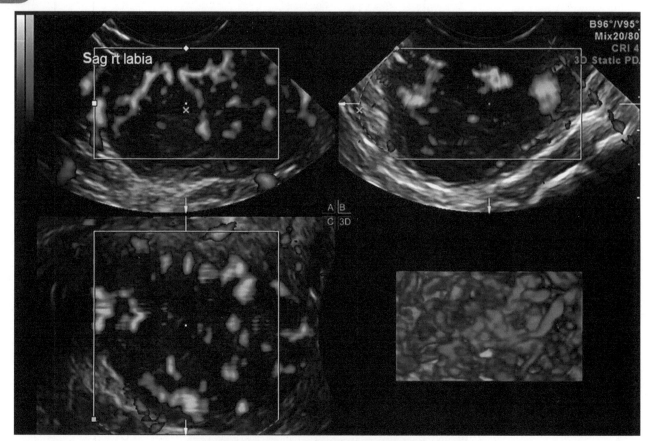

Fig. 92

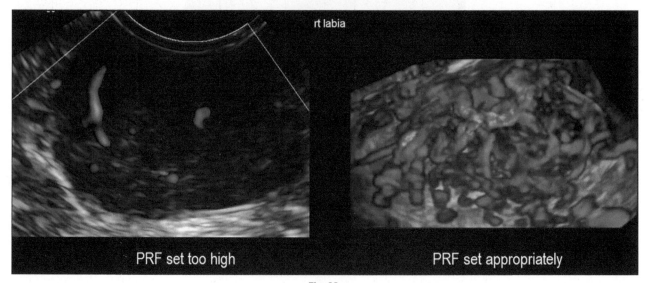

Fig. 93

CASE 42, FIGURES 94 AND 95

15. Fig. 94. With the 5–9 MHz endovaginal transducer placed transperineally at a 90-degree angle to the table on the posterior vaginal wall in a transverse plane, this anal sphincter complex (ASC) image was obtained. At what level of the ASC is this?
    a. Proximal
    b. Mid
    c. Distal

16. Fig. 95 demonstrates the 3D volume set on the same patient as Fig. 94. The very small center reference points (CRPs) through which the red and light blue lines on the planes intersect indicate the same center (green arrows) of all three orthogonal planes. The CRPs can be moved by the examiner at the time of the exam, or post exam at the 3D workstation if the volume is saved. This will allow the examiner to choose any specific level of the entire

acquired volume and manipulate the cuts for fine-tuning or additional anatomic documentation at the areas of interest.

a. The standard acquisition plane for 3D ASC assessment is seen on the A plane, which is what cut on the patient? _____
b. The B plane is what cut on the rectum? _____
c. The C plane is what cut on the rectum? _____
d. In what direction on the A plane should the CRP be moved to visualize the proximal ASC (screen right, screen left, screen top, or screen bottom)? _____

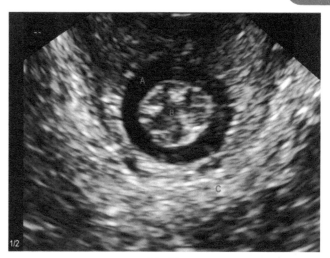

Fig. 94

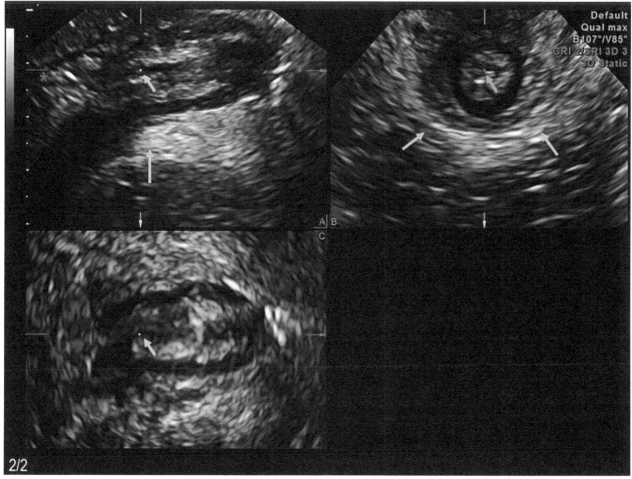

Fig. 95

CASE 43, FIGURE 96

17. Fig. 96 includes sagittal and transverse endovaginal images of the uterus of a 26-year-old woman with menorrhagia or abnormal uterine bleeding. Color Power Doppler was initiated to demonstrate uterine vascularity. Before you assess the exam vascularity, consider the normal uterine vessel branching pattern.

Normal uterine vessel branching direction is dependent on which branch is assessed relative to the endometrium. The primary uterine artery branches along the peripheral uterus as arcuate vessels ("arc" around the periphery) and are parallel to the endometrium. These branch into the radial arteries that "radiate" into the myometrium and are perpendicular to the endometrium. These branch into the spiral arteries, which approximate the endometrium also in a perpendicular approach. Normal visible sonographic vascularity at the endometrial–myometrial interface is never parallel to the endometrium.

Fig. 96. Is the peri-endometrial vascular pattern parallel or perpendicular to the endometrium *in this patient?* _____

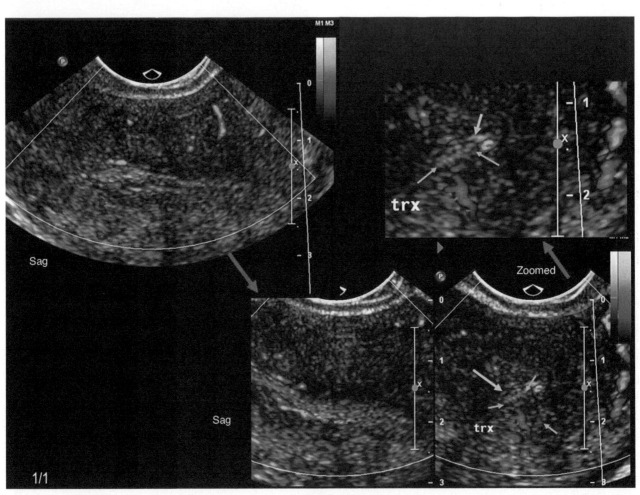

Fig. 96

CASE 44, FIGURE 97

18. In contrast, Fig. 97 demonstrates a uterine transverse cut of a larger endometrial lesion that is isoechoic to the myometrium *on another patient* who presents with menometrorrhagia or abnormal uterine bleeding. In this case, the Color Power Doppler vascular pattern is not entering centrally into the lesion but is seen along the periphery of the lesion. The endometrium is proliferative in appearance with the compressed basal (gold arrows) and functional (red arrow) layers surrounding the lesion except at the base attachment (blue lines). Remember, a myoma will typically demonstrate peripheral flow, whereas an endometrial polyp will demonstrate central flow. What is your diagnosis?

a. Intramural leiomyoma
b. Large endometrial polyp
c. Subserosal leiomyoma
d. Endometrial hemorrhagic clot
e. Submucosal leiomyoma

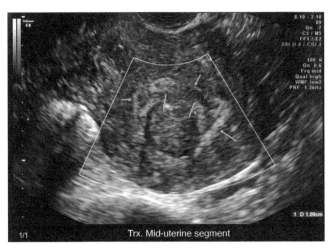

Fig. 97

CASE 45, FIGURE 98

19. Fig. 98 demonstrates a transverse cut of the mid-internal anal sphincter (IAS) on two separate patients using a 4–8 MHz endovaginal transducer. Describe the location of the IAS defect in each image as related to the hands of a clock.
    a. Image A _____
    b. Image B _____
20. Which image demonstrates elevation of the central mucosa—A, B, or both? _____
21. Which image demonstrates a more complete view of the pubovisceral muscle complex? _____
22. If the exams of Fig. 98 had been performed using a 6–12 MHz transducer, would the image resolution be worse, the same, or better? _____

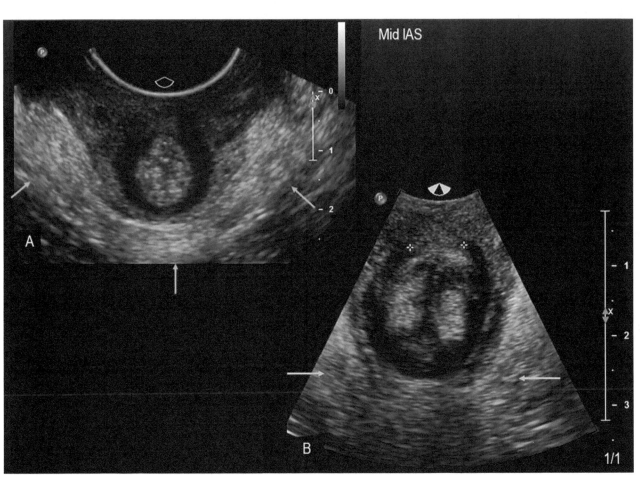

Fig. 98

CASE 46, FIGURE 99

23. Fig. 99 demonstrates the midsagittal image of the urethra using a transperineal 5–9 MHz endovaginal transducer with the screen top left image at rest and screen top right image with the patient at maximum Valsalva. A Valsalva maneuver may present a better view of the pelvic floor integrity. Screen bottom is a short video clip of a normal patient performing a Valsalva maneuver. Which of the following is the noted anatomical change?
    a. The urethral neck opens with Valsalva.
    b. The urethra demonstrates minimal bladder movement with Valsalva.
    c. The urethra demonstrates an extreme posterior/inferior change with Valsalva.
    d. The urethra demonstrates a dramatic reduction in anteroposterior diameter of the urethral/bladder neck with Valsalva.

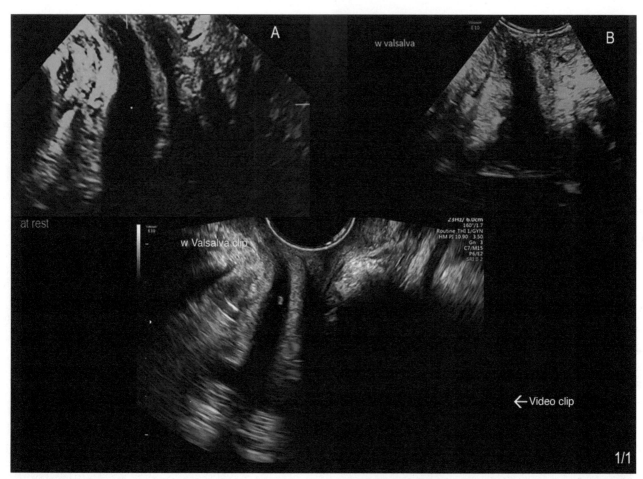

Fig. 99

CASE 47, FIGURE 100

24. Fig. 100 is an abnormal 2D transperineal axial image of the mid-internal anal sphincter (IAS) using a 6–12 MHz endovaginal transducer on a 66-year-old patient with anal incontinence. Answer the following:
    a. Describe the disruption of the IAS in terms of a clock, from _____ to _____ o'clock (OC).
    b. Is there elevation of the central mucosa toward the defect? Yes or No_____
    c. Does the anterior perianal tissue demonstrate a typical symmetric and homogeneous echo pattern? Yes or No _____

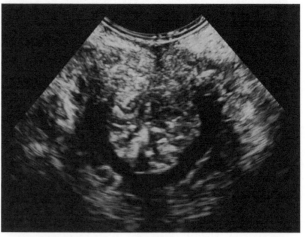

Fig. 100

CASE 48, FIGURE 101

25. Fig. 101 is a transperineal 3D volume set of the urethra using a 6–12 MHz endovaginal transducer. When a 3D volume sweep is done, the screen top left image demonstrates the sweep plane. After the acquisition is made and the volume set is present, the examiner can move the center reference point (CRP) to bring all three planes to any area of interest in the volume. To where has the CRP been moved?
    a. To the middle of the mid-urethra
    b. To the middle of the distal urethra
    c. To the middle of the proximal urethra

26. The three orthogonal A, B, C planes *of the urethra* (Fig. 101) on the volume set are which of the following:
    a. Transverse, sagittal, coronal
    b. Coronal, transverse, sagittal
    c. Sagittal, transverse, coronal
    d. Transverse, coronal, sagittal
    e. Sagittal, coronal, transverse
    f. Coronal, sagittal, transverse

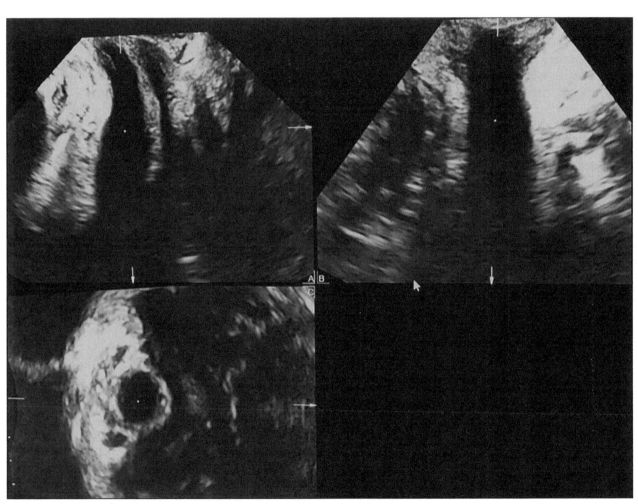

Fig. 101

CASE 49, FIGURE 102

27. Fig. 102 is a transperineal midsagittal real-time *video clip* with Valsalva of the pelvic floor anatomy using a 6–12 MHz endovaginal transducer on a 63-year-old patient with a history of a suburethral sling who now has urinary retention. The sling is visualized as an L-shaped echogenic focus as if looking into it on end (white arrows). The proximal urethra is widened but is abruptly not visible at the sling level. Additionally, the bladder (gray line) is markedly enlarged, especially noticeable on the video clip. The gold arrow is pointing to the most distal aspect of the urethra visualized. Consider the following anatomic changes *with Valsalva*:

  a. Does the urethral neck widen or close? _____
  b. Does the bladder prolapse posteriorly or inferiorly or both? _____
  c. Does the distal urethra come into view? _____
  d. Is there evidence of an enterocele at maximum Valsalva? _____
  e. Does the sling appear to compress the distal urethra? _____

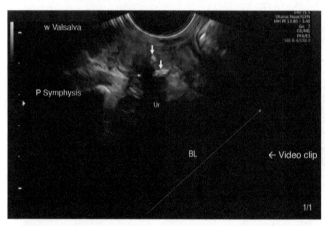

Fig. 102

CASE 50, FIGURE 103

28. Fig. 103 is a transperineal midsagittal real-time *video clip* with Valsalva of the pelvic floor anatomy using a 6–12 MHz endovaginal transducer on a 69-year-old patient who has anal incontinence. Her bladder volume post void residual (PVR) measured 153 cc.

  a. Does the bladder have normal contour? _____
  b. With Valsalva, in what direction does the bladder prolapse? _____
  c. Is there evidence of an enterocele at maximum Valsalva? _____

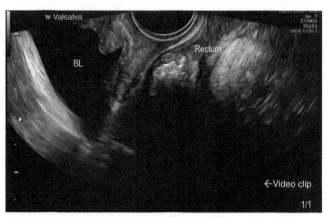

Fig. 103

CASE 51, FIGURES 104–108

29. Figs. 104–108 are images of a 42-year-old woman who is 6 weeks s/p transvaginal hysterectomy presenting with continued bright red vaginal bleeding. All images are endovaginal (EV) using a 4–8 MHz EV transducer. The right ovary is normal in appearance at the right lower quadrant and is not demonstrated here. The general survey demonstrates thickening of the vaginal cuff with increased vascularity, as seen in Fig. 104 which is a midline sagittal cut with Color Power Doppler.

Figs. 105 and 106 are the same parasagittal cuts that are left of midline, one with and one without Color Power Doppler. The plane is at the lateral edge of the vaginal cuff. In Fig, 106, structure A is the left tube, B is the left ovary, and C is the vaginal cuff.

Which of the structures has vascularity extending closest to the transducer—A, B, or C? _____

30. Fig. 107 is a Doppler color flow image of the same patient created with the transducer turned 90 degrees (transverse) from Fig. 106, which is a Color Power Doppler flow pattern. Fig. 108 is labelled. Consider the vascularity of the left tube.

  a. Is it in communication with the cuff? _____
  b. Is it in communication with the left ovary? _____

The inferior aspect of the left tube appears to be surrounded by the left lateral aspect of the cuff and adjacent to the normal left ovary. Color Power Doppler of the tube appears in communication with the vaginal cuff, as identified on all Doppler images including Figs. 104, 106, 107, and 108. Fig. 107 demonstrates extension of the left tube Doppler color flow vascularity to the edge of the cuff which was thought to be the source of the patient's bleeding.

Surgical release of the left tube from the cuff was performed and the vaginal bleeding resolved.

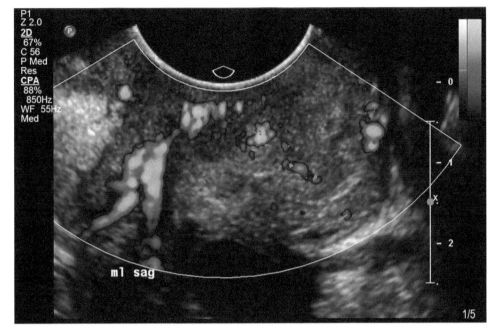

Fig. 104

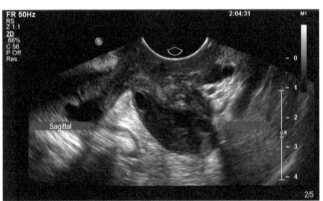

Fig. 105

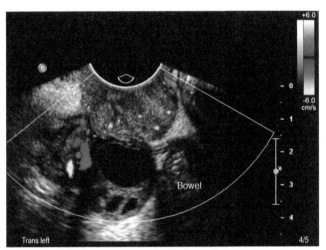

Fig. 107

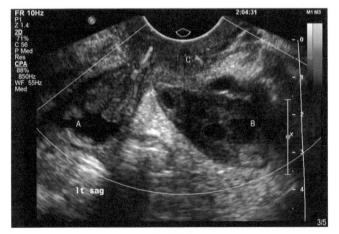

Fig. 106

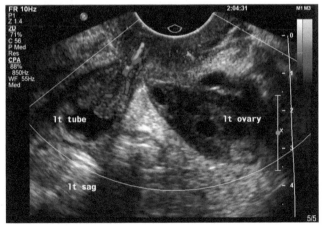

Fig. 108

CASE 52, FIGURES 109 AND 110

31. Fig. 109 is a 3D volume set of the uterus to assess the intrauterine device (IUD) location. The planes are labelled A, B, and C (white arrow at the center of the quadrants). The center reference points (green arrows) are placed on the mid-stem of the IUD and seen at the center of the three orthogonal images. What are the individual planes of the uterus?

    a. Image A _____
    b. Image B _____
    c. Image C _____

32. Which of Fig. 109 orthogonal images was the 3D sweep plane—A, B, or C? _____

33. Which plane shows the entire IUD—A, B, or C? _____

34. Which plane provides the most confidence about determining whether the IUD is present within the central cavity? _____

35. In Fig. 109, what is the gold arrow pointing at? _____

36. Fig. 110 is the C plane of the 3D volume set that has been taken out of context and rotated upright on the Z-axis. Look at the *entire* IUD. Is the entire IUD located within the central cavity? _____

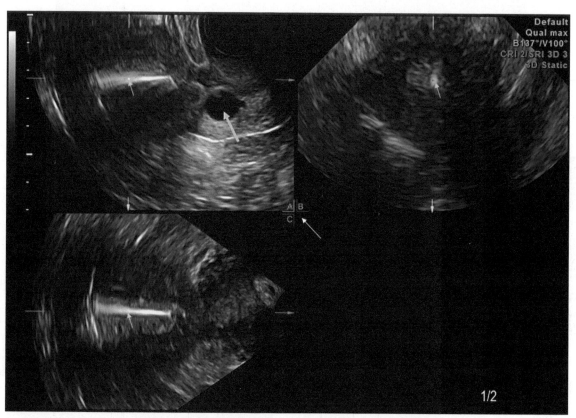

Fig. 109

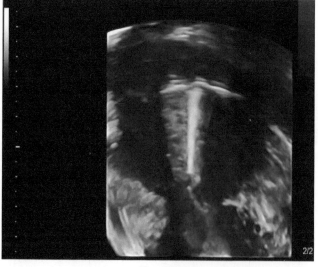

Fig. 110

CASE 53, FIGURE 111

37. Fig. 111, using a 5–9 MHz endovaginal transducer, demonstrates a rotated C plane of a 3D volume set on another patient with an intrauterine device (IUD) where the device is in the appropriate location. The stem is not seen in this image; however, the acoustic shadow posterior to the IUD stem *is* seen (as the black portion of the image, gold arrow). If the examiner parallel shifts through the 3D volume, the stem would be seen; however, the arms would likely not be seen on that cut. Two representative images should be presented if unable to visualize the entire IUD on one cut. Is Fig. 111 anterior or posterior to plane in which the stem would appear hyperechoic?

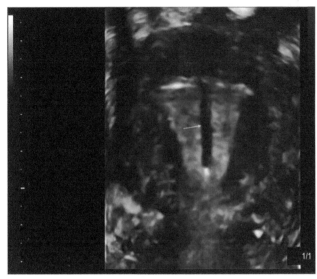

Fig. 111

CASE 54, FIGURES 112–117

38. Figs. 112–117 demonstrate the left ovary of a 39-year-old woman with left lower quadrant pain who had an ultrasound exam 4 weeks ago at an outside institution where she was diagnosed with a likely hemorrhagic corpus luteum. Review all images.

Fig. 112 is a 2D image in the transverse plane, of the left ovary, using a 5–9 MHz EV transducer. Fig. 113 is a 3D volume set where the transverse width (blue line) on the A sweep plane, the sagittal diameter (yellow line) on the B plane, and the coronal diameter (green line) on the C plane are presented. Based on these images, what does the ovarian volume measure? _____

39. Which of the following nomenclature best describes the overall appearance of the ovary?
    a. Homogeneous with multiple small anechoic structures thought to represent follicles.
    b. Diffusely homogeneous with peripheral thickened wall.
    c. Heterogeneous/complex primarily solid in appearance.
    d. Heterogeneous/complex primarily cystic in appearance.

40. The 3D volume set as seen on Fig. 113 and the rendered image of Fig. 114 indicate a thick central septum. With the center reference point (CRP) placed on the septum, and the green line of reference brought down through the septum, notice that the B plane appears as a solid ovarian component, which represents the septum (as if looking into the septum from the side).

The rendered image also demonstrates the septum; however, if the CRP were to be moved on the C plane to the central hypoechoic area in that plane instead of *on* the septum, there would be a portion of the septum that does not extend all the way across on the rendered image, indicating connectivity between the two major ovarian segments. The CRP should be moved to reflect all areas of pathology on every 3D volume set. Cut-by-cut slicing (parallel shift) through the planes will give the examiner an appreciation of the entire volume changes. Tomographic ultrasound imaging (TUI) would also provide a global cut-by-cut presentation. Notice (Fig. 113) that with the CRP (white arrow) moved *to the* septum on the A plane, B plane lies *on* the septum.

Color Power Doppler (Figs. 115–117) indicates a diffuse flow pattern around and within the ovarian parenchyma, including the septum. Multiple spectral waveform resistive indices (RIs) were taken at various locations of the ovary. A typical ovary has an RI of 0.6–0.7, but normal is considered above 0.4, although some prefer to use 0.5 as the threshold for normal.

Figs. 116 and 117. From the indices at the top right of the Doppler waveform images, what are the three RIs obtained for this exam? _____

Doppler spectral waveform indices make more sense to the examiner if one thinks about how vascular changes occur in certain disease entities. The *mechanism* for this kind of a change in Doppler spectral RI of the abnormal ovary is associated with vessel layers. Formation of the three layers of developing blood vessels results in changes in elasticity/recoil during the cardiac cycle. With neoangiogenesis, the middle layer lags in the normal quick formation such that the recoil during diastolic blood flow abnormally changes the cyclic velocities. With malignancy, diastolic flow is higher, making the systolic/diastolic waveforms more similar and the RI is reduced.

This phenomenon can occur not only in the rapidly growing vascularity of a malignant lesion but also in the common benign condition of a normal corpus luteum, which consistently has a low RI; therefore, a hemorrhagic corpus luteum can also appear quite abnormal in echo pattern with low RI; therefore, it may raise suspicion for a neoplasm, but a follow-up exam of a hemorrhagic corpus luteum will change in appearance over time and appear quite different, if not completely resolve within 6–8 weeks.

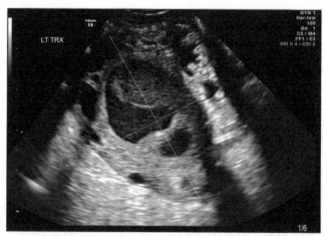

Fig. 112

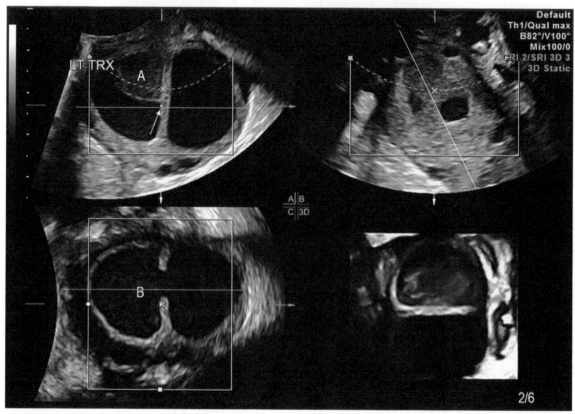

Fig. 113

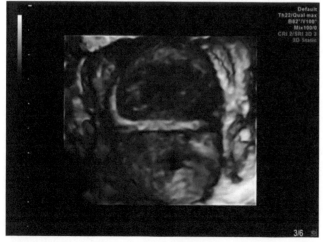

Fig. 114

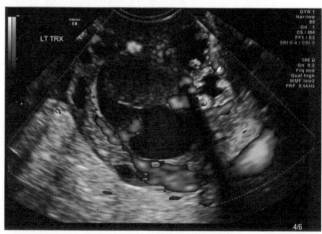

Fig. 115

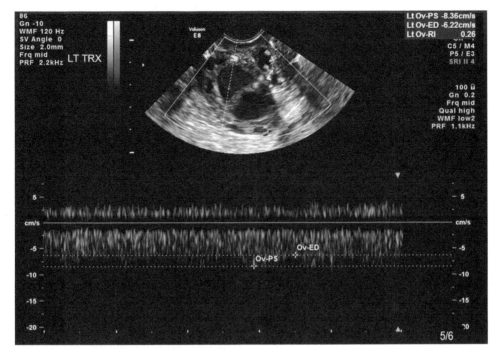

Fig. 116

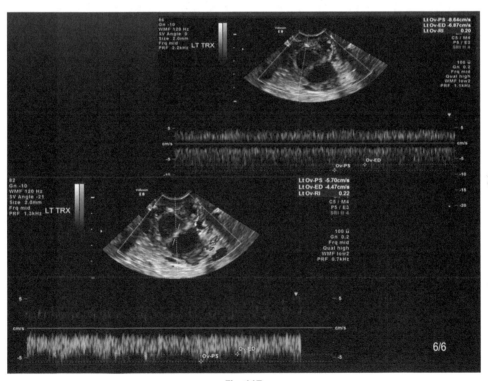

Fig. 117

CASE 55, FIGURES 118 AND 119

41. Figs. 118 and 119 (video clip) demonstrate the sonographic appearance of mesh within the pelvic
floor in a patient with a history of urinary incontinence. The purpose of this case is not to locate the
mesh level relative to surrounding anatomy, but to
demonstrate its appearance. The single 2D image
(Fig. 118) and a video clip saved from the exam
cine loop (Fig. 119) are presented using a 5–9MHz
endovaginal transducer. Using a transducer with
lower frequency such as a transabdominal transducer can image mesh, but it will appear as a thick
hyperechoic curvilinear band with poorer resolution of the actual mesh. Using a transducer with
the highest frequency can make a big difference in
resolution of the net-like appearance of the mesh
(Fig. 119 video clip).

Note that the focal point, which is the point of
convergence of the multiple beams of focused
sound coming out of the transducer, is seen along
the left side of Figs. 118 and 119 (gold arrows). It is
at the level of the mesh, which will maximize resolution of the mesh. The computer does not "know"
at what level the area of interest is during an exam;
so, the examiner should be moving the focal zone
to the level of interest throughout the exam.

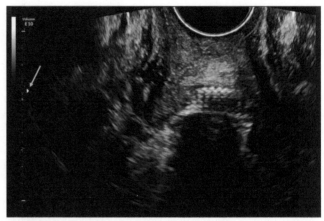

Fig. 118

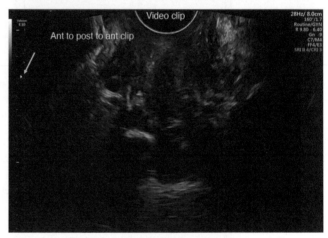

Fig. 119

Case Reviews 56–74

TOPIC 4, FIGURE 120

1. Fig. 120 Topic: Basic 3D Instrumentation

Multiplanar views, in this case of the uterus (labeled A, B or C at the image center; gold arrow), represent the three orthogonal planes surrounding a center reference point (CRP) within a 3D volume set. A is the acquisition sweep plane, B is perpendicular to the A plane at the CRP (white arrow), and C is coronal to the A plane at the CRP. On the A plane, the curved green line of reference (LOR) can be brought to an area of interest as if looking from above into the anatomy below the LOR. This can be changed by the examiner to approach the area of interest from any direction. The volume set can also be manipulated post exam at a workstation.

The "A" plane, seen at the upper left quadrant of the 3D volume set image, is the acquisition plane determined by the examiner. In the middle of the image is a CRP that demonstrates the center of the volume area of interest (white dot; white arrow).

The "B" plane is a vertical cut 90 degrees (perpendicular) to the CRP of plane A and is seen on the upper right quadrant of the 3D volume set image. In the middle of the image is the CRP that demonstrates the center of the volume area of interest (red dot; white arrow).

The "C" plane is a horizontal (coronal) cut 90 degrees to the CRP of plane A and is seen on the lower left quadrant of the 3D volume set image. In the middle of the image is a CRP that demonstrates the center of the volume area of interest (light blue dot; white arrow).

The bottom right quadrant is the location for the 3D rendered image, which is determined by the operator using various instrumentation tools, especially the LOR.

Since the 3D volume exists, any "slice" of the anatomy can be pulled out of context by parallel shifting through the volume set; therefore, it can be post-processed at a workstation. By appropriate placement of the above settings, the uterus can be seen in the sagittal, transverse, and coronal planes with an upright 3D rendered image.

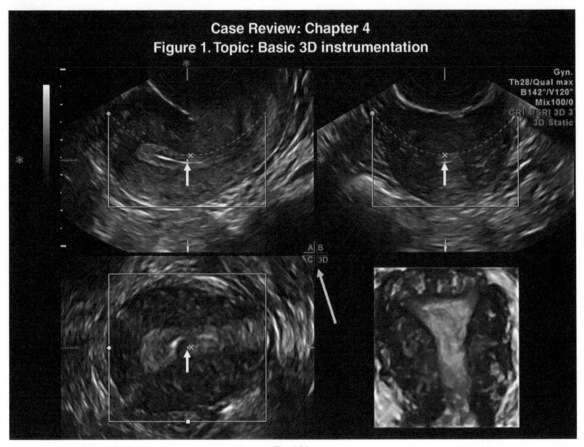

Fig. 120

CASE 56, FIGURE 121

2. Fig. 121 is a transperineal midsagittal image of the urethra at rest using a 5–9 MHz transducer. The top of the screen is inferior and screen left is anterior. The urethra is measured from the mid-bladder/urethral neck interface to the most distal visualized urethral mucosa. If it cannot be measured in one line, another can be measured and added to the first, as is seen on Fig. 121.

a. What is the urethral length of this patient? _____

b. On this image, each line-to-line distance measures 1cm. What is the urethral anteroposterior (AP) neck measurement (yellow line)? _____

c. To what is the gold arrow pointing? _____

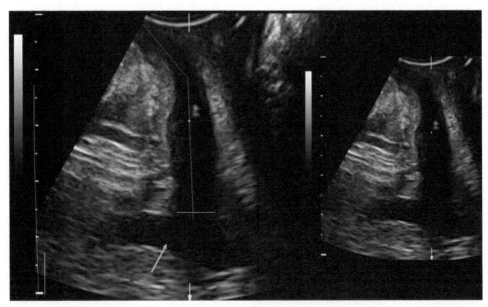

Fig. 121

CASE 57, FIGURE 122

3. Fig. 122 is a transperineal midsagittal image of the urethra at rest (A) using a 5–9 MHz endovaginal (EV) transducer and at maximum cough stopped from a cine loop (B). It demonstrates the greatest posterior movement of the urethra on this patient with minimal but reduced size in neck AP diameter (gold arrow). Using the calipers on a frozen image allows post-exam measurements of any structure. What does the AP urethral bladder neck measure at maximum cough? _____

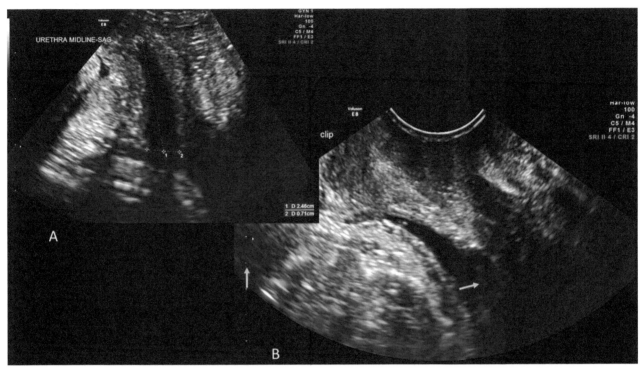

Fig. 122

CASE 58, FIGURE 123

4. Fig. 123 demonstrates a normal midsagittal urethra using a 5–9 MHz EV transducer at the perineum where a manual trace measurement calculates the urethral length. If the ultrasound system has this capability, it is the most useful in measuring curved structures such as the urethra.
   a. Is the length normal? _____
   b. Is the focal zone setting (white arrow) at an appropriate level to demonstrate the urethral neck? _____

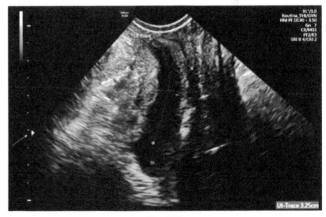

Fig. 123

CASE 59, FIGURE 124

5. Fig. 124 is an image of the normal internal anal sphincter (IAS) using a 6–12 MHz EV transducer placed perpendicularly at the posterior vaginal wall in a transverse plane. At what level is the cut—proximal, mid, or distal? _____

6. Is the posterior vaginal wall imaged? _____

7. At what anatomic structure is the focal zone indicator placed along the side of the image?
   a. Vaginal wall
   b. Puborectalis aspect of the pubovisceralis muscle (PVM) complex
   c. Lateral aspect of the PVM complex
   d. Central mucosa of the IAS

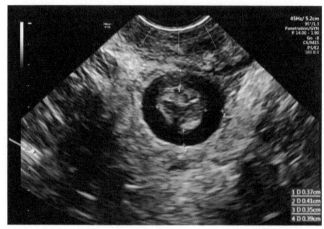

Fig. 124

CASE 60, FIGURE 125

8. Fig. 125 is performed to assess the intrauterine device (IUD) location. Screen left includes the uterine C plane taken out of a 3D volume set and rotated upright on the Z-axis. Which of the levels on the sagittal image (screen right) is the correct plane depicted on the C plane—1 or 2? _____

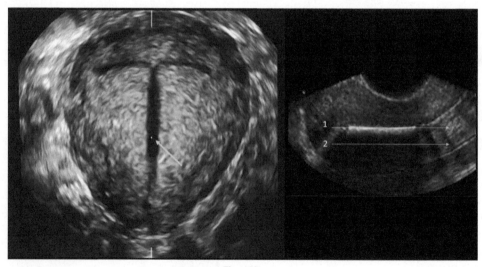

Fig. 125

CASE 61, FIGURES 126–128

9. Figs. 126–128 represent a case illustrating how correct use of the line of reference (LOR) in a 3D volume set can help to solve an issue that is otherwise nearly impossible in 2D imaging alone. Fig. 126 is a transabdominal 3D volume set done in search of a lost IUD with a concomitant 29 weeks 1d gestational age (GA) intrauterine pregnancy (IUP). Though this is a gyn case series, utilization of 3D imaging to find a lost IUD, with or without a coexisting pregnancy, is a challenge the gyn imaging specialist will likely encounter.

The patient was not experiencing any discomfort, but a previous first-trimester exam suggested its location at the lower uterine segment (LUS). Once the IUD location was suspected as remaining present within the LUS on 2D imaging, the 3D volume set was performed to confirm the IUD location relative to the fetus.

The CRP placement (red arrows, Fig. 126) is near the edge of, but not *on*, the IUD and is seen at all three orthogonal planes. In fact, the only quadrant where the IUD is clearly seen is the left lower quadrant C plane, but its relationship to the fetus cannot be seen. Notice that the 3D LOR (curved green line) is above the IUD area of interest (too high) on A and B planes, making the (screen lower right) rendered 3D image of Fig. 126 useless by including all the anatomy from the CRP level to the LOR.

What is the distance from the IUD to the edge of the fetal head, even though it globally appears "directly adjacent?" _____

In Fig. 127, by bringing the CRP to the IUD and the green LOR down to just above the IUD on A and B planes, the directly adjacent IUD location relative to the fetal head (gold arrow) is now recognizable within the medial wall of the myometrium. Fig. 128 is the 3D rendered IUD rotated upright using the Z-axis knob, but it is the volume set that reveals the relative structures.

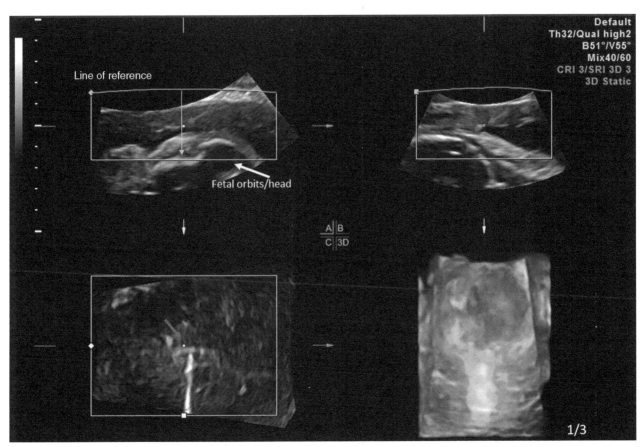

Fig. 126

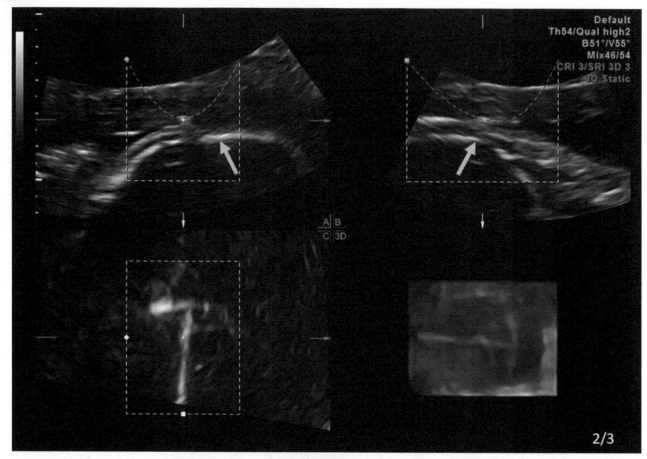

Fig. 127

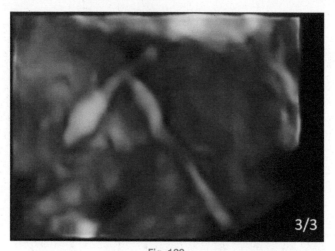

Fig. 128

CASE 62, FIGURES 129–131

10. Figs. 129–131 demonstrate transperineal transverse images of the anal sphincter complex (ASC) using a 6–12 MHz EV transducer on a patient in a great deal of pain following a history of a traumatic vaginal delivery. In these cases, the transperineal exam requires an extremely delicate touch with minimum pressure of the transducer placement on the perineum.

Normally, the transducer in a transverse position, placed at the posterior vaginal wall and angled inferiorly to superiorly, depicts the ASC near the transducer on the screen with the posterior vaginal wall appearing homogeneous and only a few millimeters in thickness. Little pressure of the transducer is needed.

In this case, the transducer contact pressure was reduced even more to demonstrate true perianal postpartum trauma swelling.

Fig. 129. Using calipers on the side of the first image, what is the distance from the transducer to the rectum in this case (red arrow to red arrow)? _____

11. Fig. 129 is at a different ASC level than Fig. 130, though both images are transverse cuts. Though the IAS is not ideally seen in either image, it is because emphasis for these images was placed on demonstration of the superficial abnormal perianal tissue.

    a. Which image demonstrates the external anal sphincter (EAS) level—Fig. 129 or Fig. 130? _____

    b. Which image demonstrates the PVM complex—Fig. 129 or Fig. 130? _____

12. With Figs. 129 and 130, both on Fig. 131, describe the perianal tissue (measured by red arrows) between the transducer and the rectum using appropriate sonographic descriptive nomenclature.

    a. Shape _____
    b. Size _____
    c. Echo pattern _____
    d. Color Power Doppler pattern _____

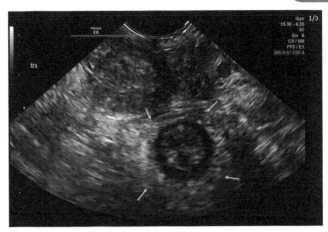

Fig. 129

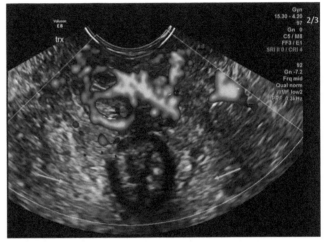

Fig. 130

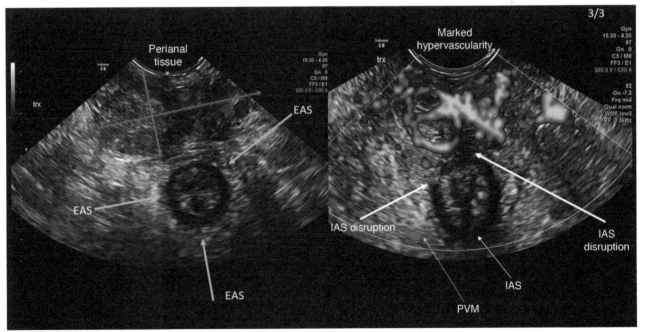

Fig. 131

CASE 63, FIGURES 132–134

13. Figs. 132–134 represent the 3D ultrasound exam that was performed on a patient who was thought to have expelled her IUD and subsequently had another inserted. Following placement of the second IUD, she began experiencing deep pelvic pain.
    a. Fig. 132. Does the 3D volume set demonstrate an IUD stem within the central cavity? _____
    b. Is the green line of reference on the A plane of the 3D volume set placed correctly to most optimally visualize the stem on the rendered image? _____
    c. Of note, however, is that the 3D rendered image (Fig. 132, bottom right of the volume set) demonstrates an additional abnormal hyperechoic structure at the lower uterine segment (LUS; green arrow). On which side of the patient is the green arrowed structure? _____
14. This case exemplifies how important moving the CRP to the area of interest on a 3D volume set is in detailing abnormal findings. We know from the 3D rendered image on Fig. 132 that the second area of interest is located at the left side of the LUS (green arrow). By moving the CRP to that structure (Fig. 133), one can see that it is not just a small hyperechoic focus when viewed in a different plane (A) but is actually a linear structure located within and extending beyond the wall of the uterus.

The A plane of Fig. 133 is a parasagittal cut to the left of midline through the hyperechoic focus because we took the CRP to that point; so, the green arrowed structure is not only along the left LUS posterior aspect of the uterine wall but also protrudes *into* the wall of the adjacent bowel.

Assessing a 3D volume set post exam at a workstation may further answer questions about how the examiner might have known if a sonographic focus is really the area of interest or not. How does one know that the hyperechoic linear structure seen on the B plane is where the asterisk is pointing on the A plane? _____

15. Sometimes, as in this case, each CRP may be poorly seen due to background echogenicities. Though the CRPs are very poorly seen in this volume set, they are always at the same location on all three planes. To clarify the location, there is a red asterisk on the A plane of the rotated linear structure (Fig. 133). When multiple linear interfaces are present, it can get confusing trying to determine which structure is real on the volume set planes. On the transverse B plane, is the CRP the linear focus "1" or "2"? _____

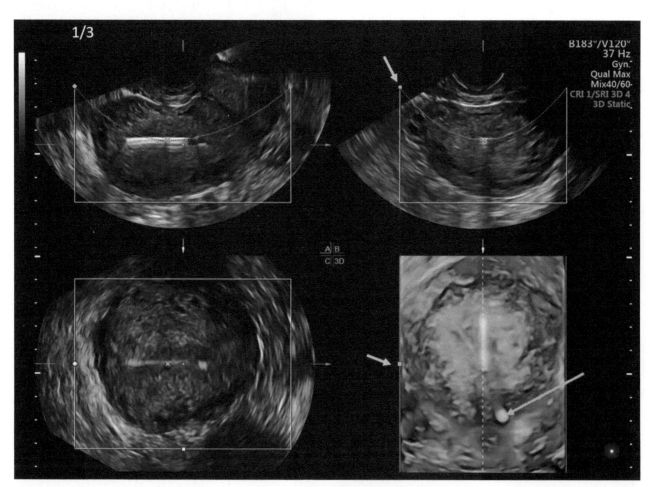

Fig. 132

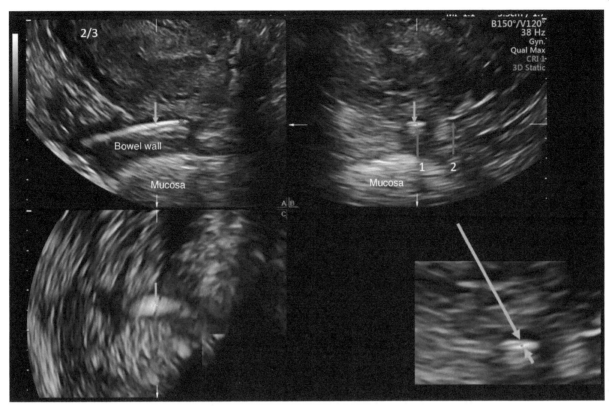

Fig. 133

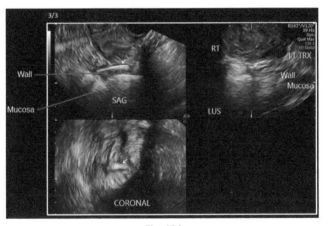

Fig. 134

CASE 64, FIGURES 135–138

16. Figs. 135–138 are those of a 42-year-old woman with menometrorrhagia, or abnormal uterine bleeding, whose last menstrual period (LMP) was 1 week ago, which would put her at the proliferative phase of the endometrial cycle. The patient came for a repeat ultrasound exam following a first exam at an outside institution. What does the endometrial thickness measure? _____

17. The normal proliferative endometrium has a distinct trilaminar appearance representing the thin consistent-throughout-the-cycle hyperechoic basal segment outside the inner gradually thickening hypoechoic functional layer. The functional layer increases in echogenicity during the secretory phase as it thickens before it sloughs off at menses. The early proliferative endometrium may only demonstrate a thin but less echogenic functional segment 1 week post menses that measures 5–7 mm.

Given her recent menses, which of the following would be the *expected appearance* of the endometrium for today's exam as opposed to what is presently shown on Fig. 135?

a. Thin hypoechoic basal layer appearance
b. Trilaminar appearance of the hyperechoic basal–hypoechoic functional–hypoechoic functional–hyperechoic basal segments
c. Homogeneous appearance of thickened isoechoic basal–functional segments
d. Thin hyperechoic functional layer with thick hypoechoic basal layer

18. What echo pattern best describes *this* endometrium?
   a. Thin basal layer appearance with thin hypoechoic functional layer
   b. Trilaminar appearance of the basal–functional–functional–basal segments
   c. Homogeneous appearance of equally thickened isoechoic basal–functional segments
   d. Thin basal layer with thick inner heterogeneous layer

19. Color Power Doppler seen on Fig. 136 demonstrates diffuse areas of vascularity within the endometrial complex. What is the most likely diagnosis as a result of this vascular pattern combined with endometrial areas of isoechoic lobular lesions measuring 7–9 mm and thin hyperechoic outer layer?
   a. Endometrial polyps
   b. Endometrial carcinoma
   c. Mid-cycle cavity fluid
   d. Submucosal leiomyomata
   e. Endometrial hyperplasia

20. Figs. 137 and 138. The same patient's previous exam report had also diagnosed a leiomyoma at the lower uterine segment (LUS)/cervical interface. A 3D volume set was performed to assess the LUS as seen on this exam. The gold arrows are pointing to the area of concern. Using correct nomenclature, describe this structure.
   a. How big is it? _____
   b. Is it round, oval, oblong, or trapezoidal? _____
   c. Is it anechoic, hypoechoic, or hyperechoic? _____

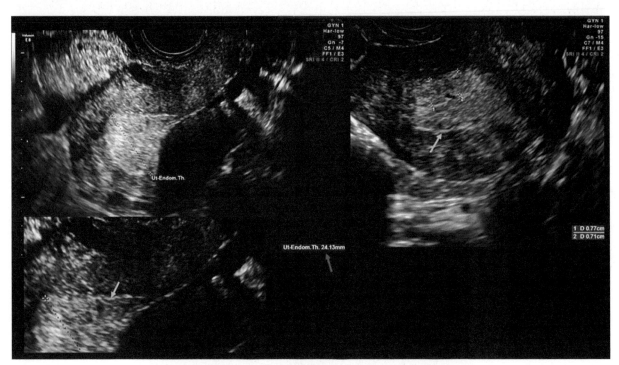

Fig. 135

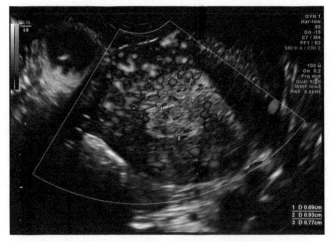

Fig. 136

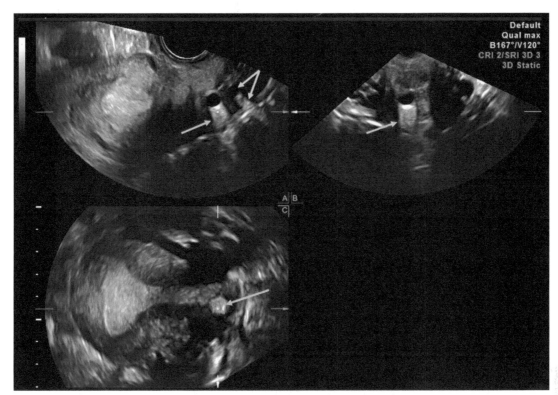

Fig. 137

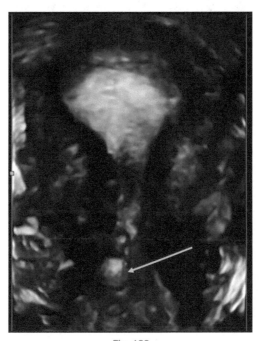

Fig. 138

CASE 65, FIGURES 139–141

21. Figs. 139–141 are those of a 30-year-old patient referred to rule out an ovarian cyst that was seen on ultrasound at an emergency room visit for pelvic pain 6 weeks ago. Transabdominal exam was performed using a 4–8 MHz transducer and a 5–9 MHz EV transducer. Her last menstrual period was 1 week ago. Both the ovaries are well visualized and appear within normal limits on this exam and are not presented. Fig. 139 is a transabdominal midsagittal image of her anteverted uterus. Fig. 140 is a 2D EV image at the same level. Which of the following descriptions best describes the arrowed structure?

a. There is an oval-shaped anechoic structure at the posterior aspect of the lower uterine segment (LUS).

b. There is a round anechoic structure at the posterior aspect of the LUS.

c. There is a hyperechoic triangular shaped structure at the posterior aspect of the LUS.

d. There is an anechoic triangular shaped structure at the anterior aspect of the LUS.

22. Fig. 141 is a 3D volume set of the uterus with the center reference point placed at the LUS/cervical interface. Is the structure midline (ML), left of ML, or right of ML? _____

23. What is the most likely etiology of this appearance?

a. Residual mid-cycle cavity free fluid

b. C-section scar

c. Degenerated leiomyoma

d. Nabothian cyst

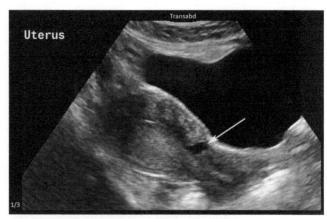

Fig. 139

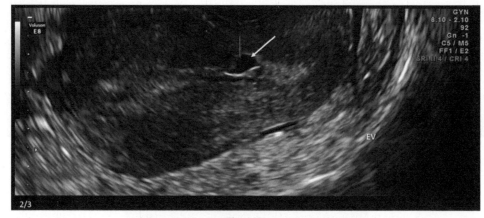

Fig. 140

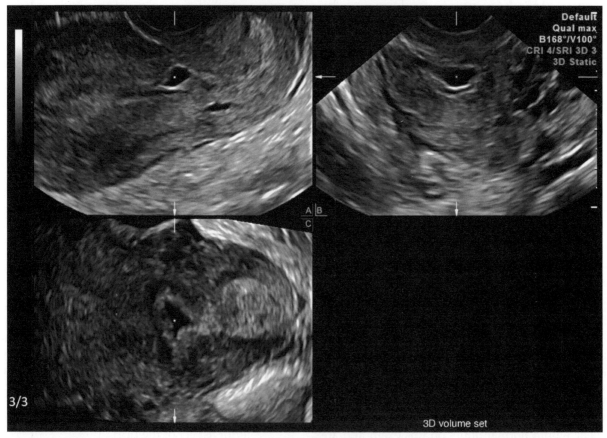

Fig. 141

CASE 66, FIGURE 142

24. Fig. 142 is a midline sagittal image, using a 5–9 MHz EV transducer, of a 65-year-old postmenopausal patient with current pessary use and a history of postmenopausal vaginal spotting. Which of the following is *not* true?
    a. The uterus is normal in length for her age.
    b. The endometrial thickness measures within normal limits for postmenopausal status.
    c. The spiral artery/endometrial interface appears normal in contour on Color Power Doppler.
    d. The anteroposterior thickness of the uterus is normal for her age and postmenopausal status.

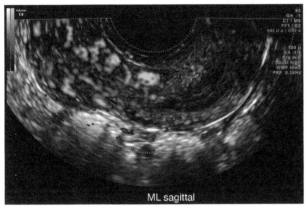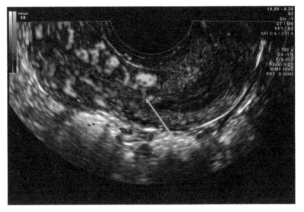

Fig. 142

CASE 67, FIGURE 143

25. Fig. 143 demonstrates transverse and parasagittal images of a patient with a bicornuate uterus who recently delivered a normal full-term newborn after a difficult pregnancy history. She absolutely did not want to become pregnant again, so her provider placed an IUD in each of the endometrial cavities. Are both stems in place? _____

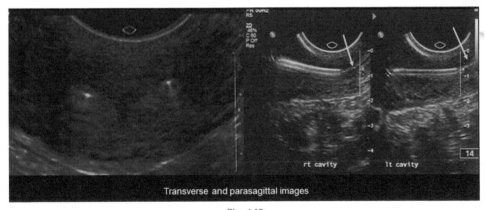

Fig. 143

CASE 68, FIGURE 144

26. Fig. 144 is a parasagittal image of the left ovary (gold arrows) of a 32-year-old who presented to the emergency room with a sudden onset of left lower quadrant pelvic pain. Her right ovary was normal and is not presented here. Which of the following group order correctly identifies the labelled 1, 2, 3, 4 structures?
    a. Iliac vessel, ovarian follicle, free fluid, corpus luteum
    b. Free fluid, corpus luteum, ovarian follicle, iliac vessel
    c. Ovarian follicle, free fluid, iliac vessel, corpus luteum
    d. Free fluid, corpus luteum, ovarian follicle, iliac vessel

27. The peripheral Doppler color flow pattern is well seen. Given the acute pain the patient experienced, what is the most likely diagnosis?
    a. Simple follicular cyst
    b. Ruptured simple ovarian cyst
    c. Ovarian malignancy
    d. Ruptured hemorrhagic corpus luteum

An acute hemorrhage has a classic latticed echo pattern that may demonstrate a layer-by-layer appearance and cause the ovarian volume to moderately exceed normal size. As the blood clots, it may have a more complex primarily solid appearance. Doppler Color Flow demonstrates a typical circumferential flow pattern around a corpus luteum, even though this was also centrally hemorrhagic, where there is no flow. Minimal peripheral anechoic intraperitoneal free fluid around the ovary suggests some degree of rupture. The patient was seen 8 weeks after this exam, and the ovary appeared normal with complete resolution of these findings.

Recommendation for follow-up, especially when the patient is young, should be conservative as hemorrhagic clots may take 6–8 weeks to resolve.

The normal mid-cycle post-ovulatory free fluid volume present within the cul-de-sac can measure up to 10 mL. With EV imaging, the field of view may subjectively appear as a voluminous presence of free fluid; however, a volumetric measurement of the fluid usually alleviates the concern.

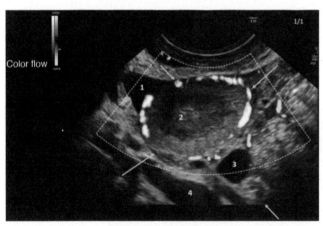

Fig. 144

CASE 69, FIGURE 145

28. Fig. 145 is another patient experiencing mid-cycle pain. Answer each of the following statements with Yes or No.
   a. The ovary contains normal follicles. _____
   b. There is moderate paraovarian free fluid present. _____
   c. The ovary contains an anechoic intraovarian lesion. _____
   d. A focal layer-by-layer intraovarian fine latticed appearance is present. _____
   e. There is acoustic shadowing distal to the transducer side of the ovary. _____

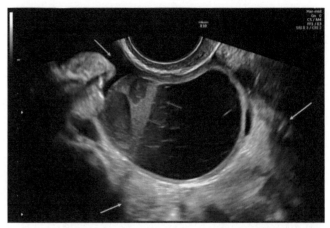

Fig. 145

CASE 70, FIGURES 146–148

29. Figs. 146–148 create an exercise related to 3D imaging instrumentation. This may seem a far too detailed example of how 3D imaging occurs; however, it demonstrates how an area may appear abnormal when it is not. When there is concern for an abnormal focal area, it can be clarified by moving the CRP to that area and be seen on all three planes.

This volume set was created using a 5–9 MHz transducer with a midsagittal sweep of the uterus and a 75-degree sweep angle.

The CRP was brought to the center of the fundal portion of the endometrium on the A plane. This can be done during or post exam at a picture archiving and communication system, also called PACS, workstation. The B plane is orthogonal to the A plane at the CRP location, creating a transverse cut. The C plane is coronal to the A plane CRP, creating a coronal cut through the uterus at the CRP location.

Note the change in echo appearance of the central endometrium/cervix interface on the C plane. Fig. 147 is the 3D rendered image for the Fig. 146 volume set. Is the circled central area that appears hypoechoic abnormal? _____

30. Fig. 148. Why, then, does not the endometrium have the hypoechoic appearance on the B plane? _____

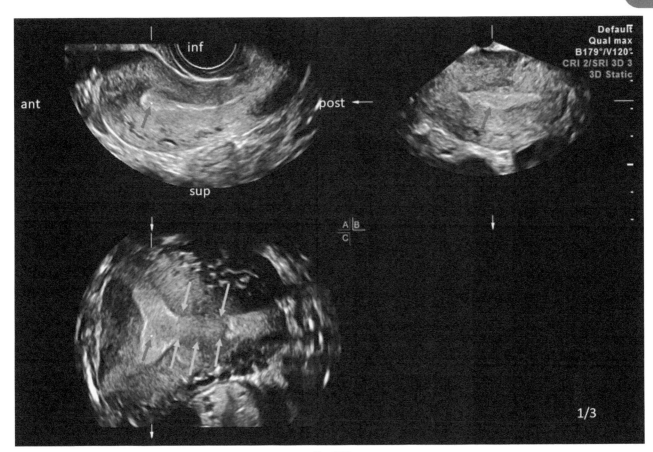

Fig. 146

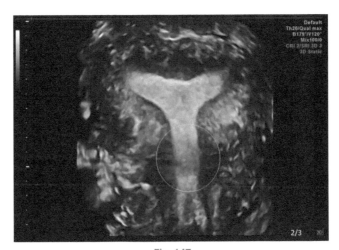

Fig. 147

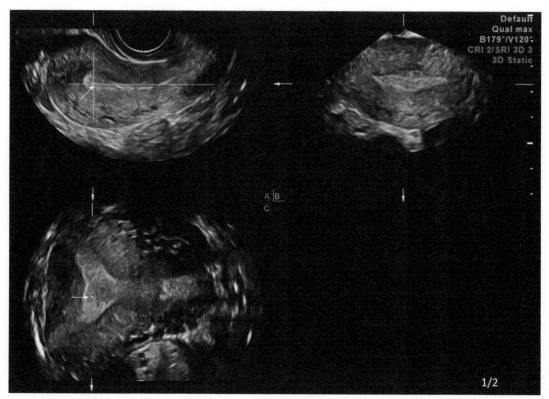

Fig. 148

CASE 71, FIGURES 149–151

31. Figs. 149–151 are transabdominal 3D images of a 14-year-old patient with gradually increasing, now severe abdominopelvic pain. She has never menstruated. The A plane of Fig. 149 is a midsagittal image of the uterus. The unusual-appearing uterus appears enveloped by a hyperechoic rim, measuring approximately 1 cm, around a curved complex hypoechoic central area with diffuse echogenic linear striations.

    The calipers of the A plane measure her vaginal length at 3.41 cm, which is undermeasured because of the transabdominal approach. It is seen on all three orthogonal planes at that location by the CRP placement of the 3D sweep (white arrows): a light yellow dot at the midsagittal vagina on the A plane, red on the transverse B plane, and light blue on the coronal C plane.

    Relative anatomy is also seen on all three planes. To what is the gold arrow pointing on all three planes? _____

32. While the length of the uterus would typically be measured on a sagittal cut, this patient's uterus is seen to be enlarged, "folded over itself," and altered in echo pattern. There is a symmetric outer hyperechoic rim that envelops a hypoechoic central component. The outer rim is thought to represent the myometrium, and the central area is thought to represent the endometrial cavity.

    Which best describes the endometrial cavity echo pattern?

a. Anechoic cavity relative to the myometrium
b. Hypoechoic cavity relative to the myometrium with diffuse linear echoes
c. Hyperechoic cavity relative to the myometrium with diffuse linear echoes
d. Isoechoic cavity relative to the myometrium

33. When the CRP is placed at the vagina on a 3D volume set (white arrows), as on Fig. 149, the B and C planes will not demonstrate the uterus, as it is off plane; so, the only image of the uterus is on plane A.

    The length of a uterus folded over itself may be inaccurately measured if it is arbitrarily measured in added segments. Fig. 150 demonstrates a manual trace through the contiguous central hypoechoic aspect of the altered A plane anatomy. This OMNI trace is made as an automatic registration walk through the 3D volume, which allows the ultrasound system to take the curved folded measurement and "stretch it out." Calipers along the side of the 3D volume A plane can then be used for measurement of the uterine cavity plus the distance for each end of the myometrium. What is the stretched uterine measurement? _____

34. Combining all this information (Figs. 149–151), it is now clear that the uterus is enlarged with the endometrial cavity markedly expanded containing a diffusely complex-appearing substance. Since she has never menstruated, which is the most likely diagnosis?

a. Hematocolpos
b. Mid-cycle free fluid
c. Endometrial carcinoma
d. Hematometra

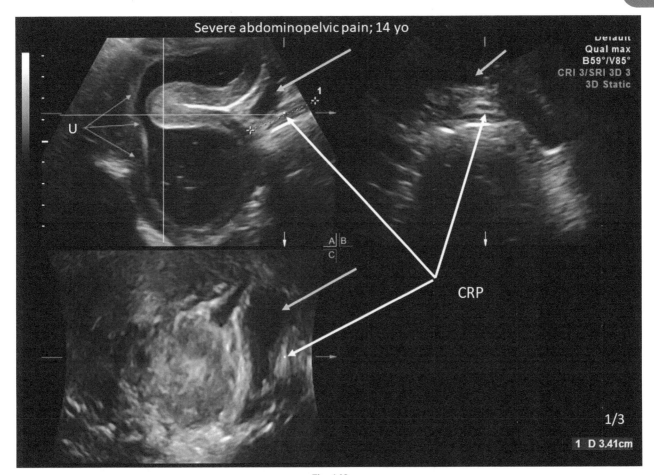

Fig. 149

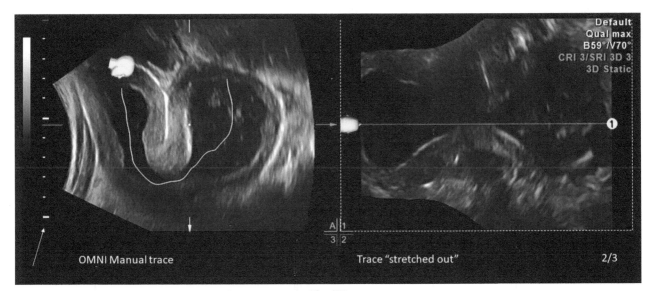

Fig. 150

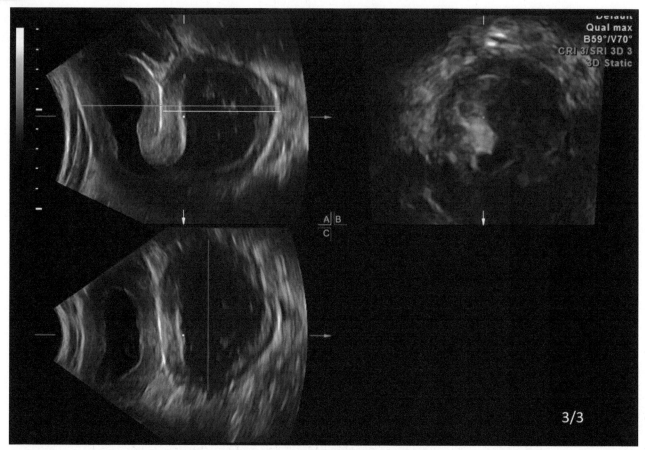

Fig. 151

CASE 72, FIGURES 152–155

35. Figs. 152–155 are those of a 43-year-old woman with a long-term history of heroin use who presented with vaginal bleeding and unrelenting excruciating pelvic pain. A 5–9 MHz EV transducer was used for the exam. Both ovaries are visualized and appear within normal limits and are not presented here. Fig. 152 is a midsagittal image of the uterus. Which of the following statements is *not* true?
    a. There is no definitive endometrial/myometrial interface.
    b. The endometrium is thickened but irregular.
    c. The myometrium appears diffusely heterogeneous.
    d. The uterus is enlarged and irregular in contour.

36. Figs. 153 and 154 demonstrate sagittal and transverse images of the cervix, which appear abnormal in echo pattern. Though the non-pregnant cervix is typically not measured, the bulbous appearance of the cervix delineates a subjectively abnormal increased size, heterogeneous echo pattern, and irregular contour. In retrospect, the calipers are undermeasuring the borders (see gold arrows).

Color Power Doppler seen on Fig. 154 portrays prominent cervical vascularity. Fig. 155 demonstrates a Doppler spectral waveform velocity of the cervical vascularity.

Which of the following additional findings is NOT present?
a. Diffuse smooth cervical contour
b. Focal cluster of punctate echogenic foci
c. Abnormal Color Power Doppler pattern
d. Abnormal cervical vascular Doppler resistive index

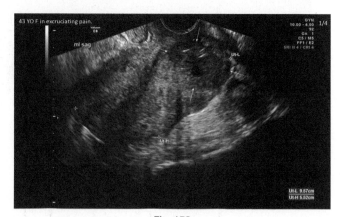

Fig. 152

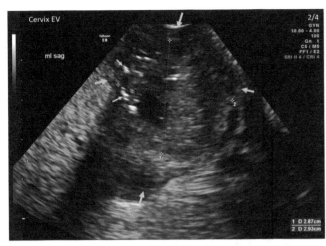

Fig. 153

Fig. 154

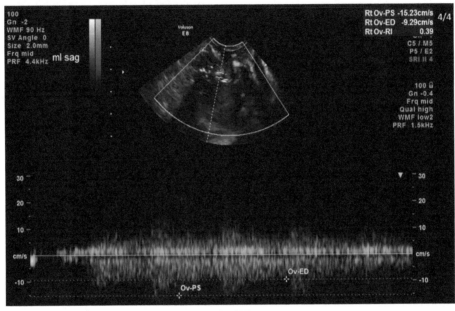

Fig. 155

CASE 73, FIGURE 156

37. Fig. 156 is a rotated C plane of a uterine 3D volume set on a patient with a history of menorrhagia, or abnormal uterine bleeding, and left lower quadrant pain. Answer the following.
   a. On which side does the uterine fundus appear abnormal in contour? _____
   b. Is the number 1 green arrowed structure contiguous or separate from the uterus? _____
   c. Is the lower uterine segment normal in echo pattern? _____
   d. Is there free fluid within the posterior cul-de-sac? _____
   e. Is the endometrium normal in appearance for a secretory phase echo pattern? _____
38. In combination, the numbered structures represent which one of the following diagnoses?
   a. Leiomyomata
   b. Left adnexal multiloculated mass

c. Abnormal endometrial thickness
d. Ovarian hemorrhagic corpus luteum components

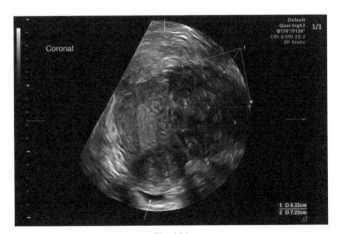

Fig. 156

CASE 74, FIGURES 157 AND 158

39. Figs. 157 and 158 are those, using a 6–12 MHz endovaginal transducer, of a 38-year-old woman who has a 10-year history of a persistent vaginal cyst with septations. She is clinically asymptomatic. About 10 years ago, it measured 1.5 cm and appeared anechoic except for several sharply defined horizontal septations. The sonographic differential diagnosis was thought to include a simple vaginal cyst and the patient has been managed conservatively. The septum remains unchanged.

At a recent exam, the lesion, located at the anterior vaginal apex, now measures 3 cm and demonstrates the presence of diffuse low-level internal echoes (Fig. 157). Additionally, a new peripheral focal hyperechoic area of vaginal thickening (green line) is noted containing several punctate echogenic foci which is thought to represent calcific infiltrations (Fig. 158).

a. (Fig. 158C) What does the maximum area of vaginal thickening measure (green line)? _____

b. (Fig. 158D) Is there no, minimal, or moderate vascularity noted with Color Power Doppler? _____

c. Does your index of suspicion for pathologic changes go up with the new presence of the calcific infiltrates? _____

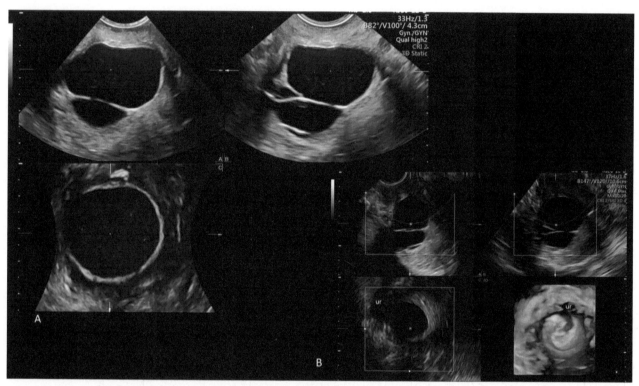

Fig. 157

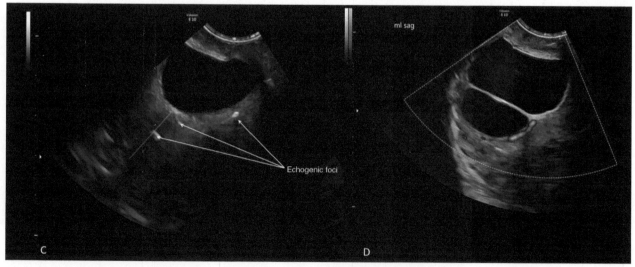

Fig. 158

Case Reviews 75–94

TOPIC 5, FIGURE 159

1. Fig. 159. Topic: Normal Endoanal 3D Image of the Distal Internal (IAS) and External Anal Sphincter (EAS)

At this axial level, the hyperechoic EAS envelops the hypoechoic IAS. Because of the biplane endoanal transducer placement *in* the rectum, the central mucosa is circumferentially displaced peripherally. Both the IAS and the EAS are intact.

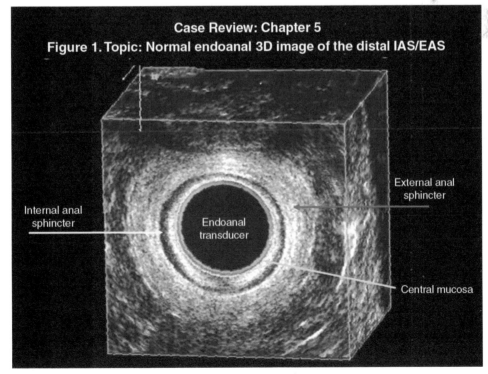

Case Review: Chapter 5
Figure 1. Topic: Normal endoanal 3D image of the distal IAS/EAS

Internal anal sphincter

Endoanal transducer

External anal sphincter

Central mucosa

Fig. 159

CASE 75, FIGURE 160

2. Fig. 160 demonstrates transperineal 3D imaging of the pelvic floor using a 5–9 MHz endovaginal (EV) transducer. The curvilinear transducer can be seen directly above the urethral and vaginal orifices at screen top (gold arrows). Which of the following structures are indicated by the gold numbers?
   a. Anterior vaginal wall
   b. Posterior vaginal wall
   c. Proximal urethra
   d. Mid-urethra
   e. Distal urethra
   f. Puboviceralis muscle complex
   g. Internal anal sphincter
   h. External anal sphincter
   i. Anal sphincter central mucosa

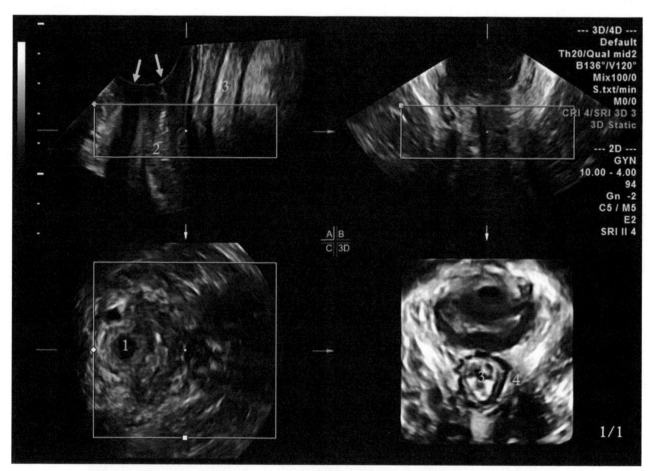

Fig. 160

CASE 76, FIGURES 161 AND 162

3. Fig. 161 is a transperineal 3D volume set of the pelvic floor using a 5–9 MHz EVtransducer. The three intersecting orthogonal A, B, C planes (at right angles to each other) are labelled at the center of the four quadrants (white arrow). A 90-degree cut at the A plane center reference point (CRP; yellow line) creates the B plane image, and the horizontal cut through the A plane from the side through the CRP (blue line) creates the coronal C plane. The various ultrasound systems will indicate on the screen where the intersecting orthogonal planes are (red and light blue side arrows). The yellow and blue lines are placed here for emphasis of those indicators.

Answer the following as related to the anatomic cuts (not the planes of the body):
   a. On what structure is the CRP placed on all three planes? _____
   b. What cut is the original sweep plane (A plane)? _____
   c. What cut is the B plane? _____
   d. What cut is the C plane? _____
4. The C plane can be isolated and then rotated upright on the Z-axis as is seen on Fig. 162. Number the following structures below in order from anterior to posterior:
   a. Puborectalis muscle complex _____
   b. Urethra _____
   c. Anal sphincter central mucosa _____
   d. Vagina _____
   e. Internal anal sphincter _____

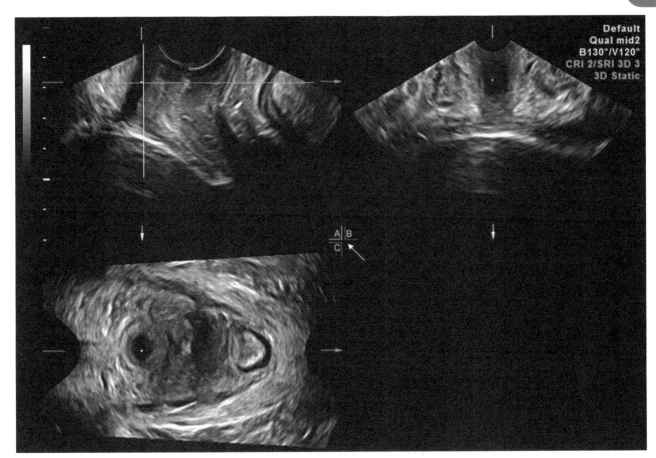

Fig. 161

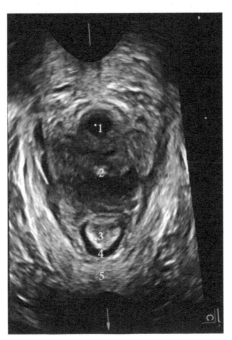

Fig. 162

CASE 77, FIGURE 163

5. Fig. 163. Compare the transperineal pelvic floor images of two patients. Like all patient populations, a large group of individuals is surprisingly varied, and imaging operator skill level and interpretation skill is crucial to optimize the assessment. The level of transducer frequency is paramount for resolution and is also operator dependent. For example, the transducer frequency of the left image is clearly a higher frequency than the right.

Poor technique may contribute to normal anatomy appearing abnormal in appearance or abnormal anatomy being perceived as normal. When interpreting transperineal pelvic floor exams, assess the images from global to specific. Of course, in the presence of an abnormality, detailed imaging at the area of interest will be necessary. Comparing the two cases, answer the following, for both the left image and right image:

a. Is the pelvic floor image symmetric? _____ _____

b. Is the urethra normal in contour?_____ _____

c. Is there evidence of urethral diverticula? _____ _____

d. Does the vagina appear as a normal smooth-bordered squared off appearance? _____ _____

e. Is there any evidence of avulsion? _____ _____

f. Is the pubovisceralis muscle complex demonstrated? _____ _____

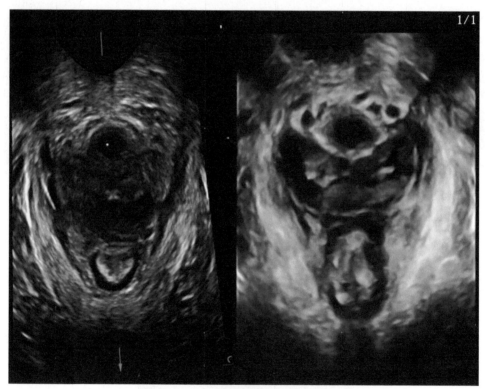

Fig. 163

CASE 78, FIGURE 164

6. Fig. 164 is a 2D transperineal image, using a 5–9 Hz EV transducer, of a 46-year-old patient with a history of mesh placement. Answer the following:

a. Is the pelvic floor anatomy symmetric? _____

b. Is the urethra normal in contour?_____

c. Is there evidence of urethral diverticula? _____

d. Does the thickened mesh have a normal bilateral smooth-bordered appearance? _____

e. Is there any evidence of avulsion?_____

f. Is the entire pubovisceral muscle (PVM) complex demonstrated? _____

g. Is the IAS symmetric in appearance? _____

h. Is the central mucosa (CM) displaced? _____

7. The operator/interpreter of the transperineal urogyn ultrasound examination should be able to look at any out-of-context isolated anal sphincter complex (ASC) transverse cut image and be able to tell:
• at what level the image was made
• whether the sphincter at that level is intact and, if not,

- at what location is it disrupted
- whether or not there is elevation of the CM toward the defect
- if, at the midlevel, the PVM complex is symmetric.

Normally, the CM is centrally situated unless there is a deviation of the surrounding IAS, which allows the mucosa to shift toward the defect. This is one of the advantages of the transperineal approach as opposed to the endoanal approach, wherein the transducer is placed into the anal canal and circumferentially compresses the CM equally by the transducer.

Which of the following is the most common plane utilized to assess the ASC?

a. Coronal
b. Sagittal
c. Axial

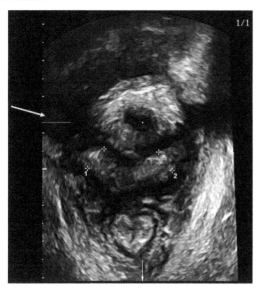

Fig. 164

CASE 79, FIGURES 165–174

Consider the following questions for Figs. 165–174, all of which are of separate patients:

a. **At what level is the ASC cut (proximal, mid, or distal)?** The proximal level appears isolated with no visualization of the PVM complex. The midlevel has distinct PVM complex inferior and lateral to the hypoechoic IAS, and the distal level hyperechoic EAS symmetrically surrounds the relatively hypoechoic IAS. The CM is seen centrally at all levels.

b. **Is it intact?** The IAS or EAS is circumferentially symmetric in the normal appearance. If not, at what level in terms of a clock is the disruption? Describe the disruption as if comparing to hands of a clock. Report, for example, that a "Disruption is noted from 10–2 OC."

c. **Is there elevation of the CM toward the defect?** Because the transducer is at the perineum and

not in the rectum, this adds a secondary finding in the event of IAS or EAS disruption as the mucosa is shifted toward the defect. Contrarily, the CM is circumferentially displaced by the transducer when placing a rectal transducer.

d. **Are the IAS and/or EAS four quadrants (12-3, 3-6, 6-9, 9-12) symmetric?** The normal IAS or EAS appears subjectively symmetric; however, measurements are comparatively the same.

e. **Does the PVM complex appear symmetric (if at appropriate level)?** The convex appearance should be bilaterally symmetric. Accomplishing this is operator dependent, not only for the 2D transperineal approach but also when creating a 3D volume set. A normal ASC can appear quite abnormally asymmetric if improperly performed.

f. **Is there evidence of a rectal/vaginal fistula?** Though this is rare, it should be assessed as part of all exams, and would be seen as a triangularly shaped extension off the IAS extending partially or all the way to the posterior vaginal wall.

8. Fig. 165. This is a transperineal ASC image.
   a. At what level is the ASC cut (proximal, mid, or distal)? _____
   b. Is it intact? _____
   c. If not, at what level in terms of a clock is the disruption? _____
   d. Is there elevation of the CM toward the defect? _____
   e. Are the IAS and/or EAS four quadrants subjectively symmetric? _____
   f. Does the PVM complex appear symmetric? _____
   g. Is there evidence of a rectal/vaginal fistula? _____

9. Fig. 166. This is a transperineal ASC image.
   a. At what level is the ASC cut (proximal, mid, or distal)? _____
   b. Is it intact? _____
   c. If not, at what level in terms of a clock is the disruption? _____
   d. Is there elevation of the CM toward the defect? _____
   e. Are the IAS and/or EAS four quadrants subjectively symmetric? _____
   f. Does the PVM complex appear symmetric? _____
   g. Is there evidence of a rectal/vaginal fistula? _____

10. Fig. 167. This is a transperineal ASC image.
    a. At what level is the ASC cut (proximal, mid, or distal)? _____
    b. Is it intact? _____
    c. If not, at what level in terms of a clock is the disruption? _____
    d. Is there elevation of the CM toward the defect? _____

e. Are the IAS and/or EAS four quadrants subjectively symmetric? _____
f. Does the PVM complex appear symmetric? _____
g. Is there evidence of a rectal/vaginal fistula? _____
h. Comment on the Color Power Doppler vascularity. _____

11. Fig. 168. This is a transperineal ASC image.
    a. At what level is the ASC cut (proximal, mid, or distal)? _____
    b. Is it intact? _____
    c. If not, at what level in terms of a clock is the disruption? _____
    d. Is there elevation of the CM toward the defect? _____
    e. Are the IAS and/or EAS four quadrants subjectively symmetric? _____
    f. Does the PVM complex appear symmetric? _____
    g. Is there evidence of a rectal/vaginal fistula? _____
    h. Comment on the Color Power Doppler vascularity. _____

12. Fig. 169. This is a transperineal ASC image.
    a. At what level is the ASC cut (proximal, mid, or distal)? _____
    b. Is it intact? _____
    c. If not, at what level in terms of a clock is the disruption? _____
    d. Is there elevation of the CM toward the defect? _____
    e. Are the IAS and/or EAS four quadrants subjectively symmetric? _____
    f. Does the PVM complex appear symmetric? _____
    g. Is there evidence of a rectal/vaginal fistula? _____

13. Fig. 170. This is a transperineal ASC image.
    a. At what level is the ASC cut (proximal, mid, or distal)? _____
    b. Is it intact? _____
    c. If not, at what level in terms of a clock is the disruption? _____
    d. Is there elevation of the CM toward the defect? _____
    e. Are the IAS/EAS four quadrants subjectively symmetric? _____
    f. Does the PVM complex appear symmetric? _____
    g. Is there evidence of a rectal/vaginal fistula? _____

14. Fig. 171. This is a transperineal ASC image.
    a. At what level is the ASC cut (proximal, mid, or distal)? _____
    b. Is it intact? _____
    c. If not, at what level in terms of a clock is the disruption? _____

d. Is there elevation of the CM toward the defect? _____
e. Are the IAS and/or EAS four quadrants subjectively symmetric? _____
f. Does the PVM complex appear symmetric? _____
g. Is there evidence of a rectal/vaginal fistula? _____

15. Fig. 172. This is a transperineal ASC image.
    a. At what level is the ASC cut (proximal, mid, or distal)? _____
    b. Is it intact? _____
    c. If not, at what level in terms of a clock is the disruption? _____
    d. Is there elevation of the CM toward the defect? _____
    e. Are the IAS and/or EAS four quadrants symmetric? _____
    f. Does the PVM complex appear symmetric? _____
    g. Is there evidence of a rectal/vaginal fistula? _____

16. Fig. 173. This is a transperineal ASC image. Note that the numbered calipers on the bottom right of the screen indicate the location of the measurement.
    a. At what level is the ASC cut (proximal, mid, or distal)? _____
    b. Is it intact? _____
    c. If not, at what level in terms of a clock is the disruption? _____
    d. Is there elevation of the CM toward the defect? _____
    e. Are the IAS and/or EAS four quadrants subjectively symmetric? _____
    f. Does the PVM complex appear symmetric? _____
    g. Is there evidence of a rectal/vaginal fistula? _____

17. Fig. 174. This is a transperineal ASC image. Sometimes when one is measuring a structure this small in the dark exam room, the more obvious borders may appear quite different when looking later at the workstation than was perceived during the exam. The solid line measurement was placed later.
    a. At what level is the ASC cut (proximal, mid, or distal)? _____
    b. Is it intact? _____
    c. If not, at what level in terms of a clock is the disruption? _____
    d. Is there elevation of the CM toward the defect? _____
    e. Are the IAS and/or EAS four quadrants subjectively symmetric? _____
    f. Does the PVM complex appear symmetric? _____
    g. Is there evidence of a rectal/vaginal fistula? _____

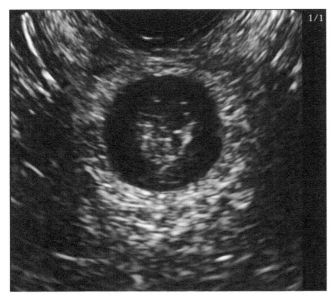

Fig. 165

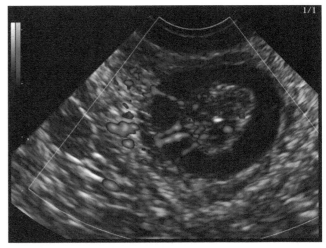

Fig. 168

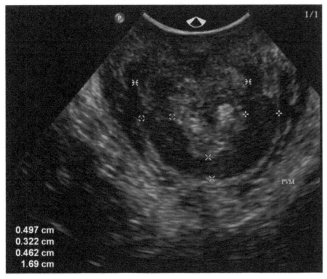

Fig. 166

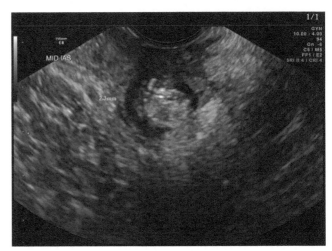

Fig. 169

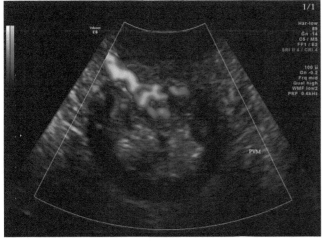

Fig. 167

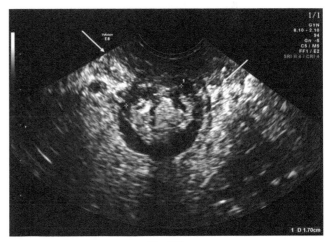

Fig. 170

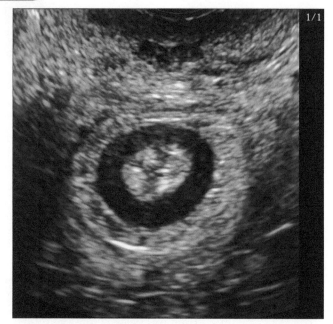

Fig. 171

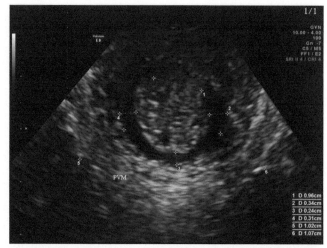

Fig. 173

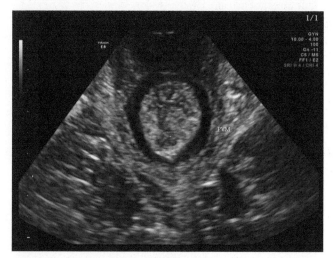

Fig. 172

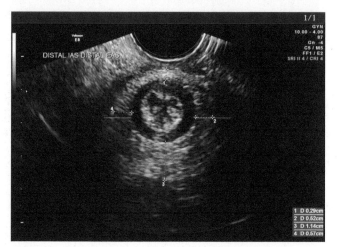

Fig. 174

CASE 80, FIGURES 175 AND 176

18. Fig. 175 is a transperineal 3D volume set of the pelvic floor of a 52-year-old patient with anal incontinence. Why is the urethra NOT visualized on the B plane when it is well seen on the other planes AND the rendered image? _____

19. Fig. 176 is the 3D rendered image of the pelvic floor 3D volume set for Fig. 175. Does the internal anal sphincter appear intact? _____

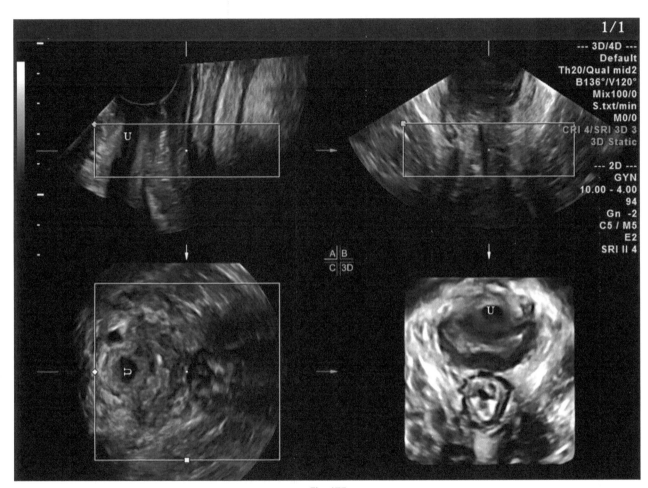

Fig. 175

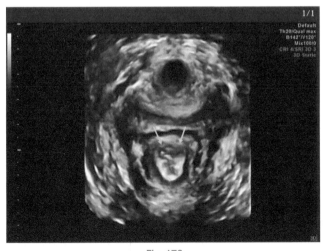

Fig. 176

CASE 81, FIGURE 177

20. Fig. 177 demonstrates sagittal and transverse post-void residual (PVR) images of a 66-year-old patient with urinary retention who self-catheterizes to empty her bladder. Note that the three dimensions are measured by the ultrasound system and the post-void residual (PVR) is calculated. Is this PVR reduced, normal, or increased? _____

21. Is the bladder wall contour smooth or irregular? _____

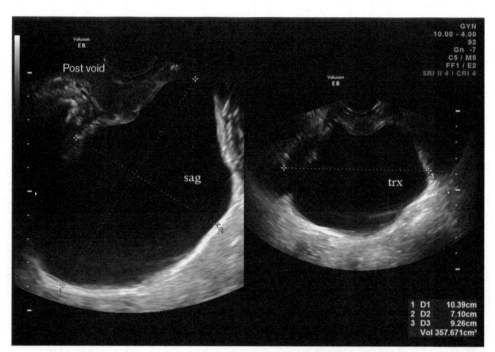

Fig. 177

CASE 82, FIGURES 178–181

22. Figs. 178 and 179 are 2D transperineal midsagittal images, using a 5–9 MHz EV transducer, of a patient who presented with difficult painful voiding. Which portion of the urethra is poorly seen?
    a. Proximal
    b. Mid
    c. Distal

23. Figs. 180 and 181 are the transperineal 3D volume sets of her pelvic floor that demonstrate how varied the anatomical appearance of the urethra can be. Note that the urethra is subjectively widened, especially at the proximal segment. Does that "widening" appear smooth or irregular in contour? _____

24. Fig. 181. On what specific structure is the center reference point? _____

25. Which of the following is the most likely diagnosis for the above findings?
    a. Urethral diverticulum
    b. Obstructed distal urethra with distal wall thickening sequelae
    c. Distal urethral abscess with proximal wall widening sequelae
    d. Cystocele

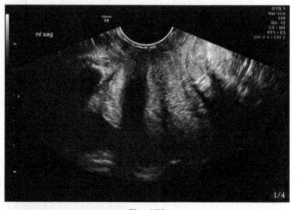

Fig. 178

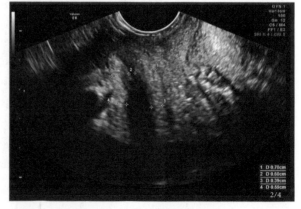

Fig. 179

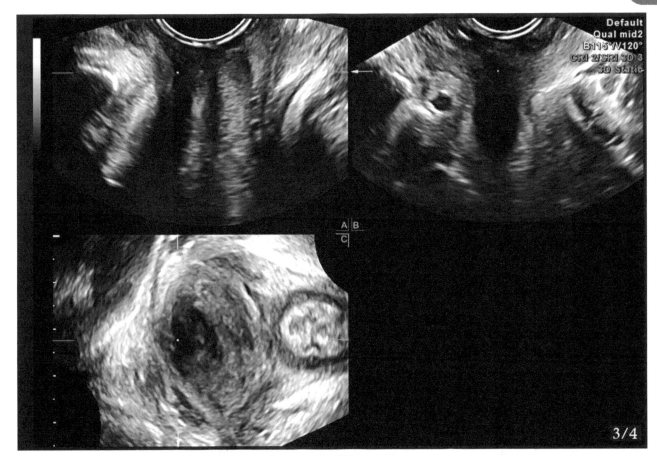

Fig. 180

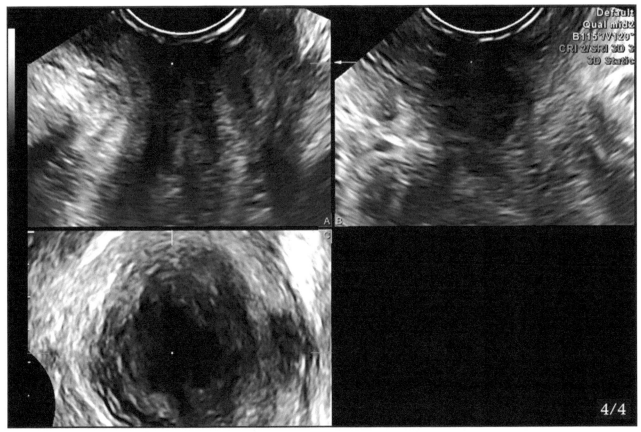

Fig. 181

CASE 83, FIGURE 182

26. Fig. 182 is a transperineal 3D rendered image of the pelvic floor using a 5–9 MHz EV transducer on a 33-year-old patient. The image demonstrates the PVM complex surrounding the anal sphincter complex. Does the PVM complex appear symmetric along the lateral mid-internal anal sphincter? _____

27. Look at the vaginal contour all the way around its circumference and look for any obvious bulging, especially at the anterior/lateral borders, which would indicate a potential avulsion. Is there evidence of pelvic floor avulsion on this single image? _____

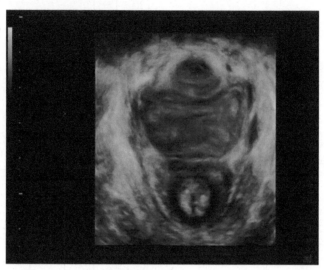

Fig. 182

CASE 84, FIGURES 183 AND 184

28. Figs. 183 and 184 are transperineal 3D volume sets of the pelvic floor using a 6–12 MHz EV transducer on a 68-year-old with urinary incontinence. The patient had mesh placed 2 years ago followed by continued urinary incontinence. The sweep plane is a midsagittal cut with the transducer placed directly at the urethral meatus. Fig. 184 is another acquisition at a slightly sharper transperineal posterior angle to improve the 3D rendered image. Note that the center reference point is placed *on* the visible mesh. Is the mesh at the proximal, mid, or distal urethral level? _____

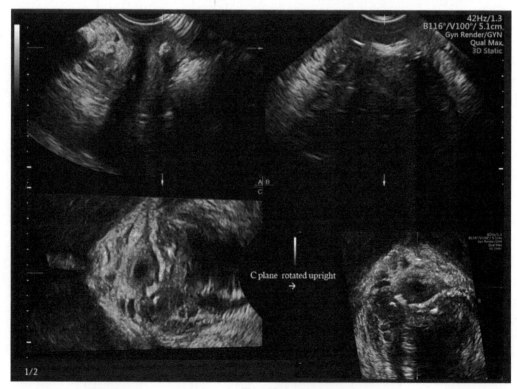

Fig. 183

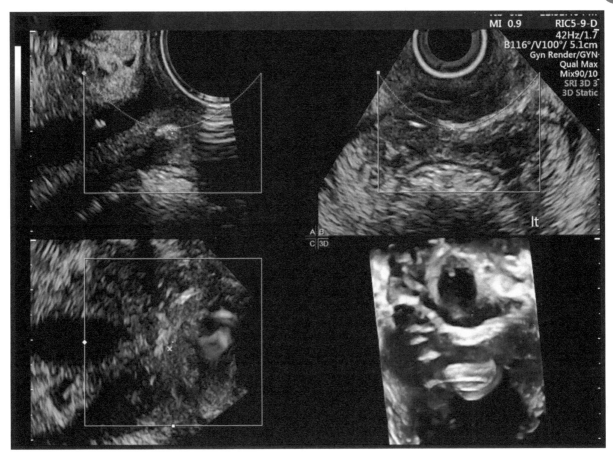

Fig. 184

CASE 85, FIGURES 185–187

29. Figs. 185–187 are transperineal images of the empty bladder, using a 5–9 MHz EV transducer, of a 69-year-old patient with a clinical history of anterior compartment prolapse that was found to be a cystocele on today's exam. An incidental finding reveals the presence of a mass within the bladder. In what aspect of the bladder is the "mass" found (superior, inferior, anterior, posterior, right, left)?

_____

30. Her bladder wall was noted to be thickened (red line, Fig. 187), measuring > 7 mm. Remember, the normal bladder wall should be < 5 mm if empty and < 3 mm if full. Hers is empty. Figs. 185 and 187 are using Color Power Doppler. Does the mass demonstrate any intralesional vascularity Yes or No? _____

31. Is the mass smooth or irregular in contour? _____

32. Fig. 185. Does the mass demonstrate posterior acoustic shadowing? _____

33. Fig. 186 is another 3D volume set of the mass with the 3D rendered image. Note that the structure can be more confidently seen as a single intrabladder hyperechoic irregular lesion. Which of the following is the most likely diagnosis?
    a. Hypervascular bladder neoplasm
    b. Avascular urethral/bladder neck neoplasm
    c. Avascular focal bladder trabeculation
    d. Avascular bladder stone

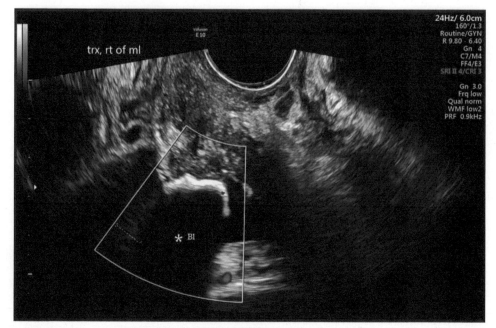

Fig. 185

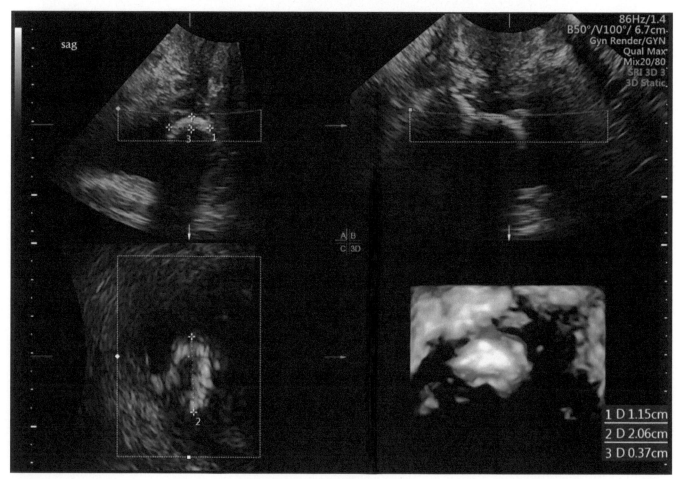

Fig. 186

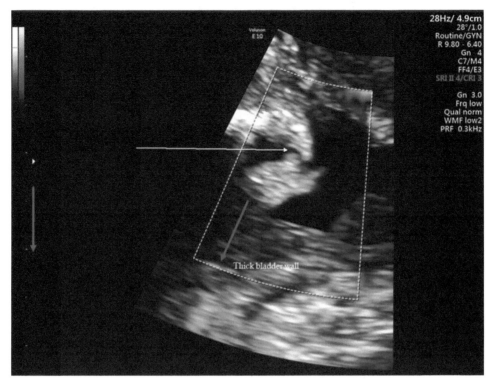

Fig. 187

CASE 86, FIGURES 188 AND 189

34. Figs. 188 and 189 are transperineal 3D volume sets of the ASC using a 6–12 MHz EV transducer. The 3D rendered image for both figures has been removed. The patient, a 40-year-old female, has a history of a wide local excision along her perineum and now experiences anal incontinence. Identify which ASC cut each of the planes represents:
    a. Plane A _____
    b. Plane B _____
    c. Plane C _____
35. The gold arrows are pointing to the CRP on Figs. 188 and 189 of all three orthogonal planes. The CRP dots in this case are difficult to see due to the echo patterns of the anatomic structures on which they are positioned, but the cross-section of the volume cuts (red and yellow lines) are extensions of the small lines at the image edges placed by the ultrasound system to delineate the intersecting planes.

    Both A and C planes demonstrate that the proximal ASC is screen left and distal ASC is screen right. The level of the B plane can be seen at the mid ASC by the bilateral appearance of the PVM complex. The PVM can also be seen (green arrows) on the A plane at the mid IAS.

By moving the CRP right or left on the volume set on either the A or C plane, one can evaluate the transverse B plane at any level.

The added subset 2D image at the bottom of screen right of Fig. 188 is placed at the same level to help compare 2D with 3D findings.

Fig. 189 is a similar 3D volume set with the CRP placed at a slightly more distal location (as seen on the A and C planes). The intersecting red and yellow lines along the edges no longer have the whole connecting lines across the image (as seen on Fig. 188). Notice that the CRP is at the distal puborectalis muscle, and the blue arrows surround the muscle now appearing as if it is "coming at you on end." The image is post-processed as Chroma. Sometimes our eyes see borders better with Chroma. Work with the one that works best for you.

The key to diagnosing ASC abnormalities is being at the best level for the B plane axial cut, from which an abnormality can be described most confidently.

As related to the B plane, does the surrounding anatomy confirm the mid ASC level? _____
36. The internal anal sphincter is not intact. From where to where is there a disruption? _____
37. Is there elevation of the central mucosa? _____
38. Is there evidence of a rectal/vaginal fistula? _____

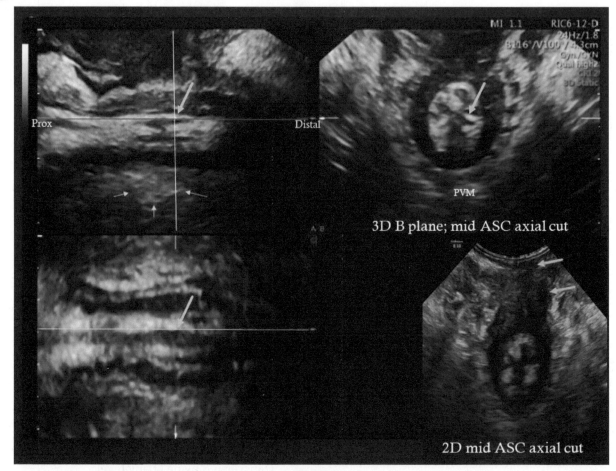

Fig. 188

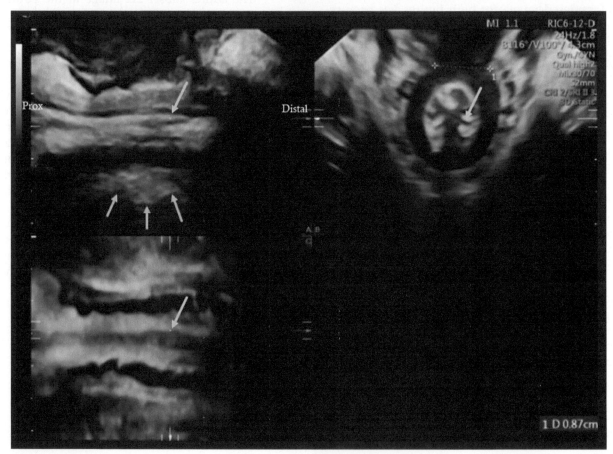

Fig. 189

CASE 87, FIGURES 190 AND 191

39. Fig. 190 is a transperineal 2D image of the pelvic floor, using a 6–12 MHz EV transducer, of a 51-year-old patient who has had a mesh *replacement* for urinary incontinence. The urethra is shown in a sagittal plane with both the original (gold arrow) and the replaced mesh (blue arrow) visualized. As can be seen, the original mesh is located mid-distally relative to the urethra and the second mesh is at the proximal-mid urethra.

Fig. 191 is the axial cut pulled out of the 3D volume set to demonstrate both mesh structures. To which does the white arrow point, the original or the second mesh? _____

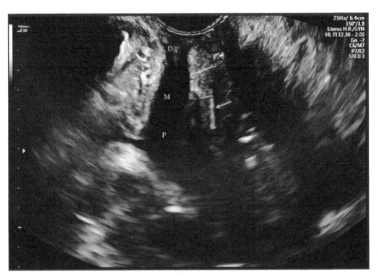

Fig. 190

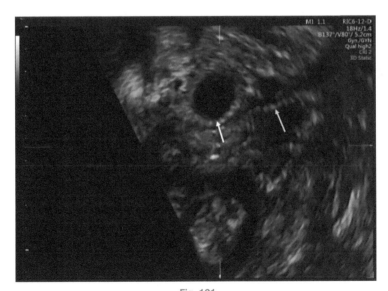

Fig. 191

CASE 88, FIGURE 192

40. Fig. 192 is a schematic of the proper endovaginal placement of a 3D biplane endocavitary transducer. After the 3D volume set is obtained, the 3D cube can be manipulated to view any axial, sagittal, coronal, and oblique views. In which of the following planes does the image (screen right) demonstrate the pelvic floor?
    a. Axial
    b. Sagittal
    c. Coronal

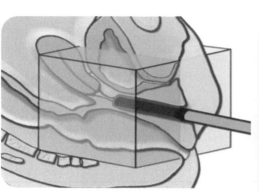

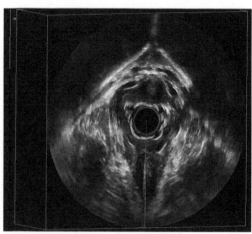

Fig. 192

CASE 89, FIGURE 193

41. Fig. 193 is an axial image of a 3D volume set of the pelvic floor using a 10 MHz biplane transducer placed endovaginally. For your orientation, the patient's left side will be at the right side of the screen and the patient's right side on the left (as if one is looking "up" the patient). The pubic symphysis, urethra, transducer (in the vagina), and the rectum have all been labeled. The blue arrow is pointing to the pubic symphysis, the yellow arrow to the urethra, and the red arrow to the rectum.

41a. Which aspect of the pubic bone complex is more echogenic, the central symphysis or the lateral rami?

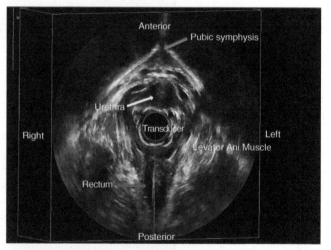

Fig. 193

CASE 90, FIGURE 194

42. Fig. 194 demonstrates a midsagittal cut of the same 3D cube volume. Labeled are the pubic symphysis, bladder, urethra, the transducer (in the vagina), and the rectum. Note the green volume box surrounding Fig. 194. If the examiner parallel shifts through this volume set, from which direction would the anatomy become visualized?
    a. Midline to lateral
    b. Lateral to midline

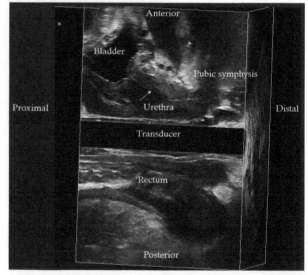

Fig. 194

CASE 91, FIGURE 195

43. Fig. 195 is an axial image of the pelvic floor using a 10 MHz biplane endocavitary transducer placed in the vagina. Identify the structures labeled A–E:
    a. Urethra ____
    b. Rectum ____
    c. Transducer ____
    d. Pubic Symphysis ____
    e. Levator Ani Muscle ____

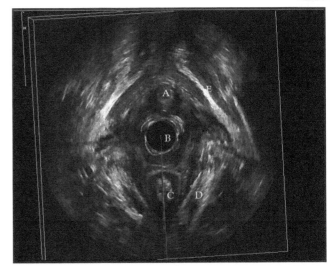

Fig. 195

CASE 92, FIGURE 196

44. Fig. 196 is a 3D axial image of the mid-pelvic floor using a 10 MHz biplane endocavitary transducer placed in the vagina of a 46-year-old female with a history of a forceps delivery presenting with complaints of dysuria, recurrent urinary tract infections, and pelvic pain for 8 months. Upon further questioning, she also complains of a vaginal bulge sensation. Her pelvic examination was nonspecific except for the presence of a palpable periurethral mass. Which of the following is the most likely sonographic diagnosis?
    a. Perirectal abscess
    b. Vesicovaginal fistula
    c. Rectovaginal fistula
    d. Urethral diverticulum
    e. Bartholin's cyst

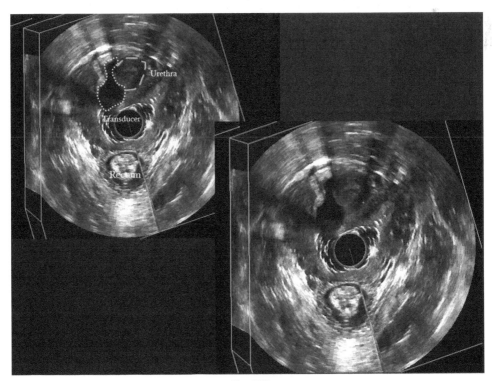

Fig. 196

CASE 93, FIGURE 197

45. Fig. 197. A 56-year-old patient with a history of several pelvic surgeries presented for evaluation because of pelvic pain. She reported a history of mesh placed in "some" of her surgeries; however, no operative reports were available. She did not tolerate a pelvic exam due to severe vaginal pain. She underwent a 3D endovaginal ultrasound exam using a 10 MHz biplane endocavitary transducer. Fig. 197 demonstrates a midsagittal view. Identify the structures labeled A–E:

a. Anterior vaginal mesh
b. Endovaginal transducer
c. Bladder
d. Suburethral sling
e. Rectum

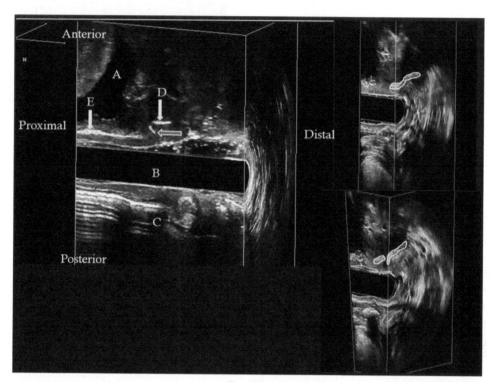

Fig. 197

CASE 94, FIGURE 198

46. Fig. 198 is an axial image of the ASC using a 10 MHz biplane endocavitary transducer placed into the rectum. Notice you are able to discern this is an endoanal ultrasound image, as compared to endovaginal, by the presence of the transducer *in* the rectum as evidenced by the round circle in the middle of the anatomy and the absence of the central mucosa except at the peripheral rim to where it has been displaced and compressed.

The transducer is placed in the rectum with the notch of the handle located anteriorly, which would make the top of the image the 12 OC segment of the distal internal and external anal sphincter level.

47. Identify the structure labeled A. _____
48. Identify the structure labeled B. _____
49. Fig. 198. Note there is a defect in the distal ASC. Which muscle is involved? ___
50. Describe the defect location as hands on a clock. The defect is seen from _____ OC to _____ OC.

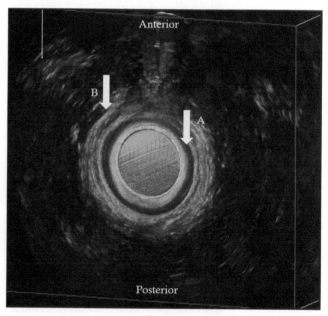

Fig. 198

Case Reviews 95–111

Outline

TOPIC 6, FIGURE 199

1. Fig. 199. Topic: Tomographic Ultrasound Imaging (TUI) of the Normal Transperineal Anal Sphincter Complex (ASC) 3D Volume Set

   TUI is the creation of operator-determined slices of a 3D volume set that can be presented into any of the orthogonal planes; so, it will start from the 3D volume set (screen left). The slices can be made thinner or thicker to view the anatomy, much like a parallel shift through the 3D volume.

   The right screen top is the midsagittal ASC image (top left) divided into axial planes, which are presented from proximal to distal. The right screen bottom takes the axial cut out of the volume set and divides it into right to left parasagittal slices. TUI is wonderful for looking globally to find the most specific area of pathology in a similar way as parallel shifting through the volume set to the appropriate level.

Case Review: Chapter 6
Figure 1. Topic: TUI of the normal transperineal anal sphincter complex (ASC) 3D volume set

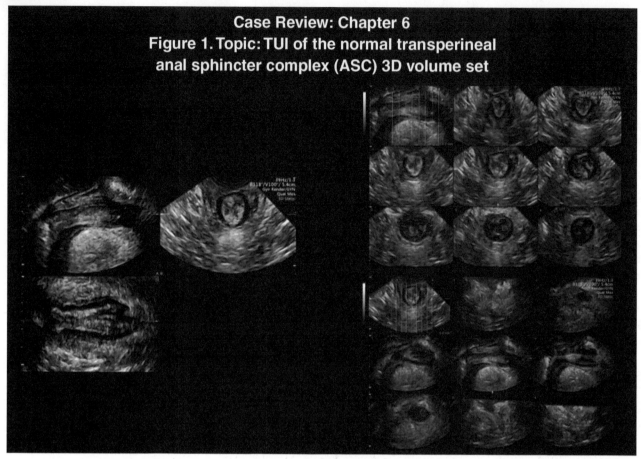

Fig. 199

CASE 95, FIGURE 200

2. Fig. 200 represents a midsagittal image of the uterus of a 22-year-old who is post menses. She was referred to follow up an "ovarian cyst" found on a previous exam 2 months ago. Her ovaries are normal on this exam and are not presented. Color Power Doppler is applied to demonstrate normal uterine vasculature. The uterine arteries branch into the arcuate arteries that "arc" along the periphery of the uterus. These branch to the radial arteries that "radiate" through the myometrium perpendicularly relative to the arcuate arteries. These branch to the spiral arteries that "spiral" toward the endometrium. As the vessels approach the endometrium, note that the normal branching vessels lie perpendicular to the basal layer of the endometrium. Screen bottom is a cross-section of the uterine vascular pattern.

Of these vessels on both images, which are the labeled structures?

a. _____

b. _____

c. _____

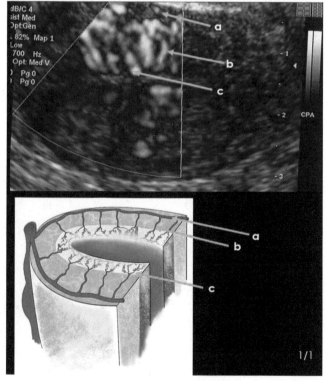

Fig. 200

CASE 96, FIGURES 201 AND 202

3. Figs. 201 and 202 are sagittal and transverse images, using a 4–8 MHz endovaginal (EV) transducer, of a 30-year-old with a history of three early pregnancy losses. She is on day 8 of her cycle. Sonohysterography was performed, but with the placement of the catheter, the saline infusion did not fill the cavity; instead, it pooled at the cervical/vaginal interface.

Which of the following descriptions best describes the uterine/endometrial vascular pattern on Fig. 201?
   a. Uterine vessels are normal, lying perpendicular to the endometrium
   b. Uterine vessels are abnormal, lying perpendicular to the endometrium
   c. Uterine vessels are normal, lying parallel to the endometrium
   d. Uterine vessels are abnormal, lying parallel to the endometrium

4. Fig. 202 is a transverse image of the uterus on the same patient. The arrows surround the transverse endometrium circumferentially. Combining Figs. 201 and 202, which of the following is true about the endometrial Color Power Doppler pattern?
   a. There is normal diffusely perpendicular vascular endometrium.
   b. There is normal circumferential intramural vascular branching pattern.
   c. There is normal peri-endometrial vessel branching pattern.
   d. There is abnormal peripheral to central vascular branching pattern.

5. Which of the following is the best sonographic diagnosis for this appearance?
   a. Endometrial polyp
   b. Endometrial mid-cycle free fluid
   c. Submucosal myoma
   d. Endometrial carcinoma

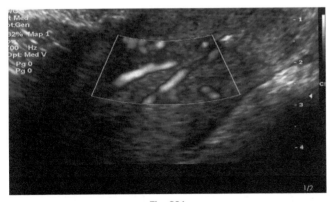

Fig. 201

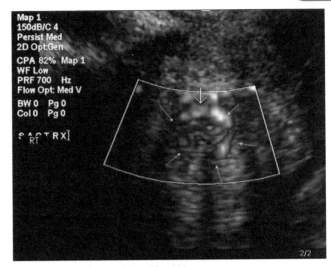

Fig. 202

CASE 97, FIGURES 203 AND 204

6. Fig. 203 demonstrates transabdominal and EV images of a 38-year-old with a 2-year history of pelvic pain. The frequency of the transabdominal transducer (top) was 4–8 MHz and that of the EV transducer (bottom) was 5–9 MHz. The left ovary was well visualized and appeared within normal limits and is not presented.

Compare the resolution of the right adnexal mass to assess the abnormal right adnexa using a lower-frequency transabdominal approach (top image) to a higher-frequency EV approach (bottom images). For example, with the transabdominal approach, the right adnexal mass appears anechoic, suggesting the presence of a simple cyst.

The volume of the ovary is increased, measuring 52.8 cc. Which of the following is the best description of the EV image of the right adnexal mass?
   a. Well-circumscribed round anechoic mass with enhanced through transmission
   b. Poorly circumscribed oval-shaped mass with diffuse low-level echoes
   c. Well-circumscribed lobular mass with dependent latticed linear echoes
   d. Endometrioma

7. Fig. 204 demonstrates Color Power Doppler application to the 3D volume set of the mass. Note that there are no vessels seen within the mass, and the 3D rendered image demonstrates vascularity adjacent to the lesion. Which of the following is the most likely sonographic diagnosis of the adnexal mass?
   a. Hemorrhagic corpus luteum
   b. Simple ovarian follicular cyst
   c. Dermoid
   d. Endometrioma
   e. Ovarian neoplasm

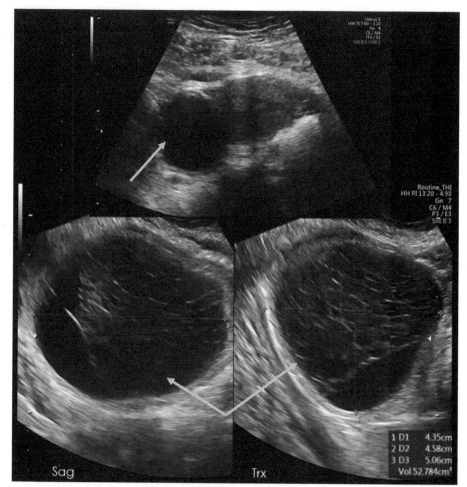

Fig. 203

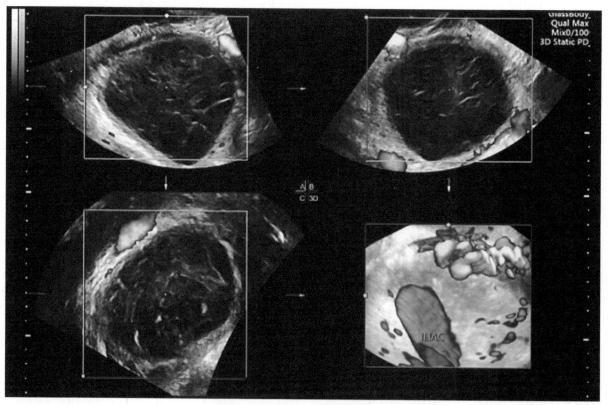

Fig. 204

CASE 98, FIGURE 205

8. Fig. 205 is a short *video clip* of a transperineal midline sagittal normal urethra with cough. Identify the labeled *directions* on the patient's body.
   a. _____
   b. _____
   c. _____
   d. _____
9. In what direction does the normal urethra move with cough?
   a. Inferiorly
   b. Anteriorly
   c. Superiorly
   d. Posteriorly

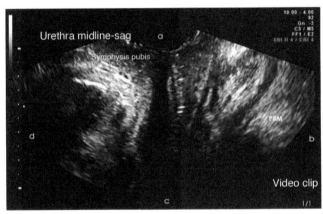

Fig. 205

CASE 99, FIGURES 206 AND 207

10. Figs. 206 and 207 are transperineal images of a 68-year-old patient with urinary incontinence. She has a history of urinary incontinence and known mesh placement for stress urinary incontinence. The top right image (Fig. 206) is her bladder and urethra at rest, and the bottom image is a frozen image of a cine loop at maximum cough. The gold arrow points to her mesh. It is located posterior to the urethra at the proximal, mid, or distal position? _____

11. The comparison of the two images demonstrates how profound an improperly supported urethra and bladder can change with cough (bottom left image). Relative to the urethra, the mesh moves completely out of the field of view with her cough, obviously not supporting the urethra. A properly placed mesh should be at the level of the mid-urethra with support, demonstrating little movement when the patient coughs. How does the urethra change with cough (blue arrow)?
    a. It opens completely
    b. It closes completely
    c. It kinks closed to a near-horizontal position
    d. It kinks closed to a near-vertical position
12. As the bladder fills and expands with nonsupport (cystocele), in what direction does it bulge?
    a. Inferiorly
    b. Inferiorly and posteriorly
    c. Superiorly
    d. Posteriorly
    e. Superiorly and posteriorly
13. Fig. 207 is a transperineal *video clip* of the pelvic floor with a Valsalva maneuver. Which of the following is *not* demonstrated?
    a. Swirling of sedentary particles in the bladder with Valsalva
    b. Inferior/posterior movement of the mesh with the bulging bladder
    c. Normal closure of the urethra with Valsalva
    d. Inferior movement of the small bowel anterior to the anal sphincter complex

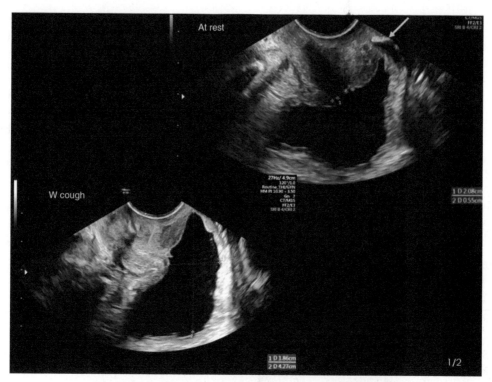

Fig. 206

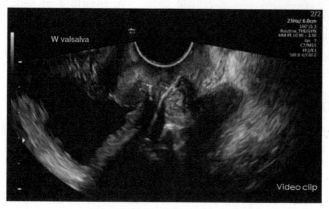

Fig. 207

CASE 100, FIGURES 208–215

14. Figs. 208–215 are those of a patient referred for pelvic fullness. She was diagnosed with bilateral ovarian cysts based on an ultrasound exam from an outside institution. Figs. 208 and 209 are ambiguous transabdominal images of complex hypoechoic pelvic masses through only a partially filled bladder. Sorting through this kind of complex findings takes patience with deliberate evaluation of anatomy. Fig. 209 is a transabdominal transverse view of what was thought to represent the left ovary (calipers). The remainder of the exam was performed with a 5–9 MHz EV transducer. Fig. 210 is a midline (ML) sagittal transperineal image of the pelvic anatomy with the transducer placed halfway into the vagina, demonstrating how far inferiorly the complex mass extends

(yellow arrows). Identify the labeled *directions* on the image of the ML sagittal cut of Fig. 210.

a. _____

b. _____

c. _____

d. _____

15. Fig. 211 demonstrates visualization of the right ovary of the same patient, appearing normal; therefore, the complex structures are likely extra-ovarian. Fig. 212 is a transverse view, ML on the patient, which is the plane where the previous exam may have perceived adjacent bilateral ovarian cysts. With the transducer turned 90 degrees and to the right through this area, as seen on Figs. 213 and 214, several of the oval-shaped nearly anechoic structures now appear directly on top of each other, suggesting the presence of

bilateral serpiginous structures folded over themselves. A measurement of the right structure width is 5.2 cm (measurement at calipers).

With a 3D sweep through this area, the volume of the tri-structured relationship can be manipulated using an OMNI view trace, as seen on Fig. 215, which additionally demonstrates all components as contiguous. The ability to trace through the curve allows the actual length to be measured (blue arrows, measure 1). Stretched out now, it measures 8.3 cm. Of the list below, what is the most logical diagnostic conclusion of this appearance?

a. Fluid-filled adjacent small bowel
b. Intraperitoneal pelvic ascites
c. Bilateral hydrosalpinges
d. Bilateral corpus lutea

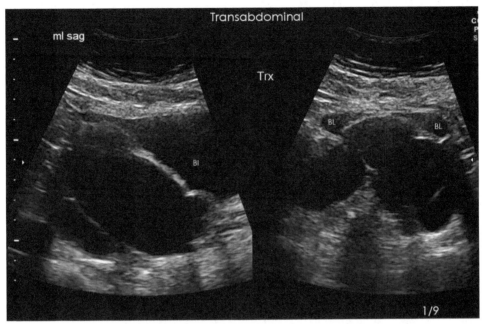

Fig. 208

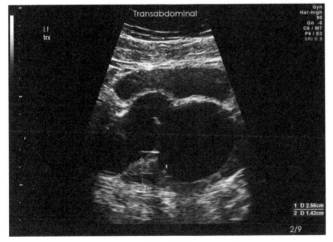

Fig. 209

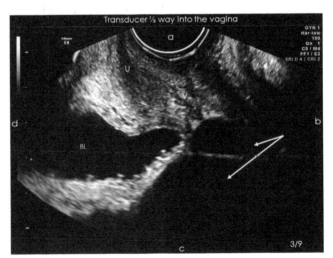

Fig. 210

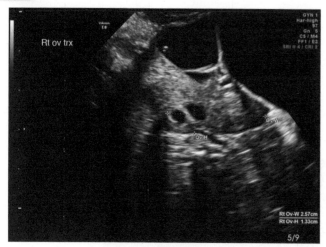

Fig. 211

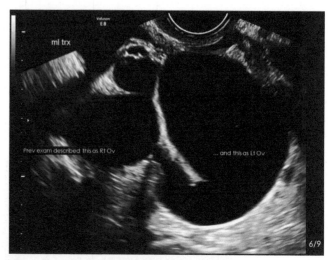

Fig. 212

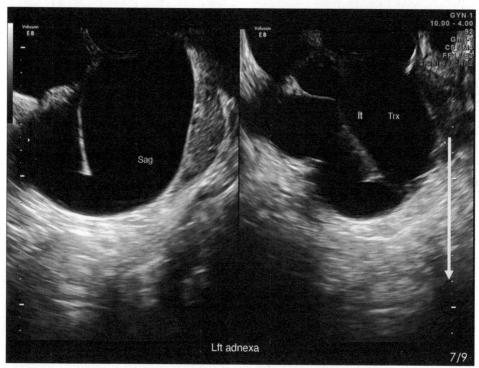

Fig. 213

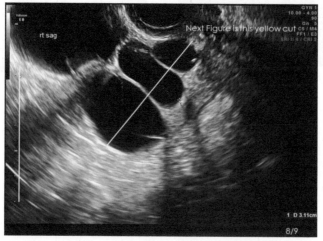

Fig. 214

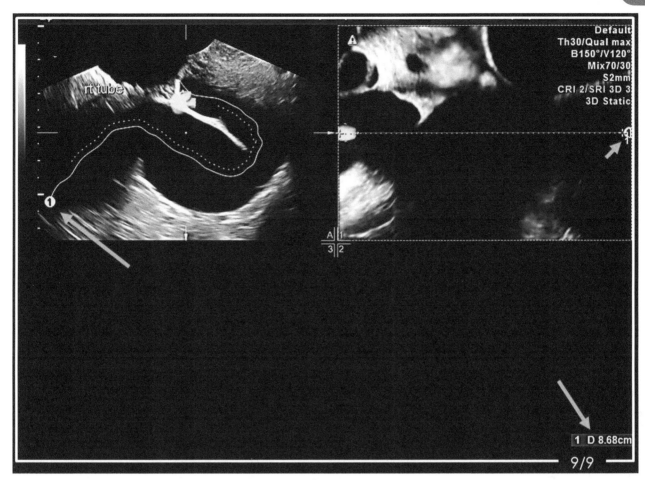

Fig. 215

CASE 101, FIGURES 216 AND 217

16. Figs. 216 and 217 demonstrate 2D versus 3D imaging to assess for intrauterine device (IUD) placement location. In what position is the uterus?
    a. AV, AF
    b. AV
    c. AV, RF
    d. RV
    e. RV, RF
17. In Fig. 216, 2D images demonstrate the stem (Image #1) and the arms (Image #2). With the 2D EV approach, and the uterine position as it is, it is certain that the IUD is in place; however, the transducer cannot be rotated to see the coronal plane. Observe the 3D volume set on Fig. 217.
    a. What is the sweep plane utilized for the 3D volume set? _____
    b. What are each of the labeled B and C planes? _____
    c. Which of the four quadrants is the entire IUD visualized? _____

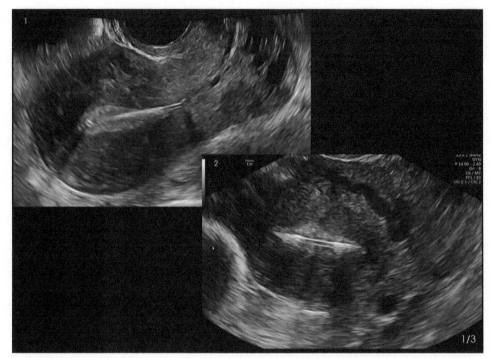

Fig. 216

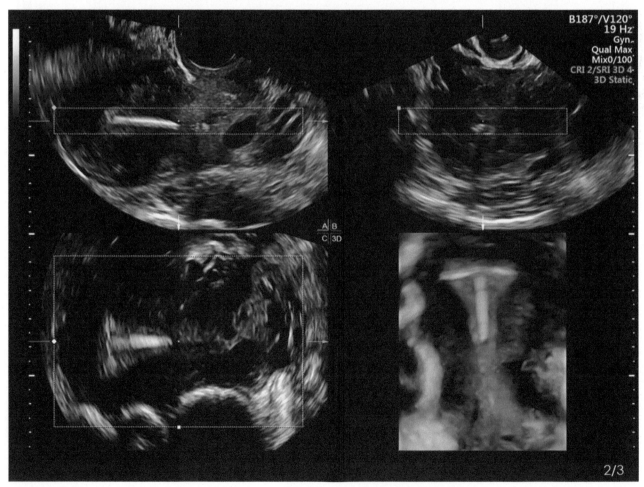

Fig. 217

CASE 102, FIGURES 218–220

18. Figs. 218–220 are those of a 35-year-old with a history of infertility. Fig. 218 presents a sagittal and transverse image of the uterus. Which one of the following statements is *not* true?
    a. The uterus demonstrates multiple submucosal leiomyomata.
    b. The functional and basal layers of the endometrium are both visualized.
    c. There is minimal free fluid within the endometrial cavity.
    d. There are several endometrial lesions seen within the endometrial cavity.

19. The 3D volume rendered image adds significant overall clarity to the finding, as seen on Figs. 219 and 220. Though the rendered image appears frozen, like a 2D image would appear, any of the A, B, or C orthogonal planes or 3D rendered image (blue arrows) can be manipulated to the most optimal positions using the X-, Y-, and Z-axis knobs. Each knob has a rotary control of a volume set image with rotation around any one of the axes' display plane to display any desired view. Additionally, the parallel shift knob can merely sweep through the volume of any plane. Remember, the center reference point (CRP) can also be moved on any plane if the volume set remains (at the time of the exam or at a workstation post exam) to obtain the most diagnostic images.

Why are the abnormal lesions *not* seen on the C plane on Fig. 219?
    a. Because the line of reference for the 3D rendered image is too anterior to the lesions
    b. Because the CRP puts the C plane at the endometrial basal layer
    c. Because the sweep angle was too narrow
    d. Because the rendered image was rotated too far on the Y-axis
    e. Because the area of interest box is too thin

20. Which of the following is the most logical etiology for the patient's infertility?
    a. Subserosal leiomyoma
    b. Submucosal leiomyoma
    c. Diffuse leiomyomata
    d. Multiple endometrial polyps

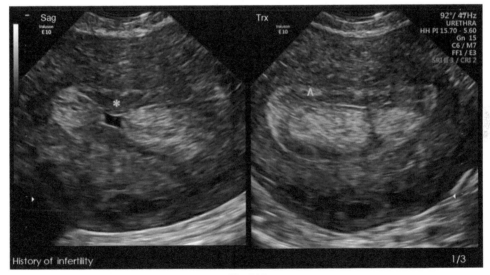

Fig. 218

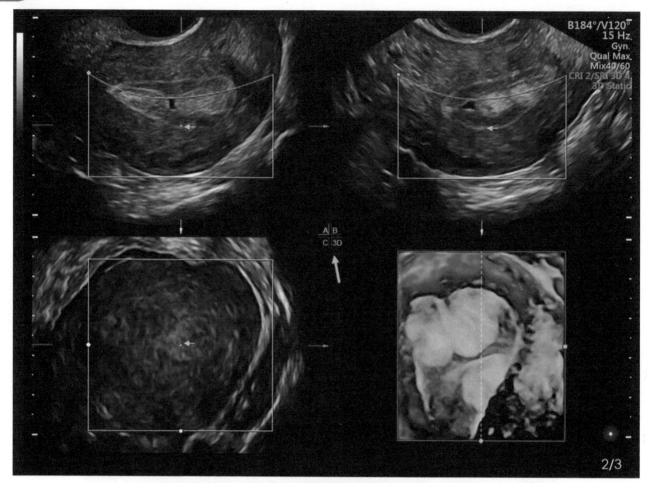

Fig. 219

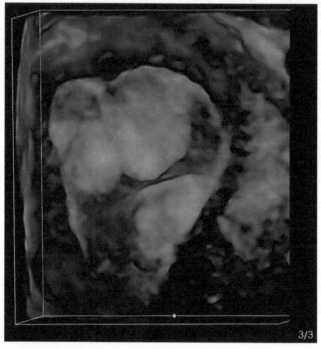

Fig. 220

CASE 103, FIGURE 221

21. Fig. 221 is a transperineal 3D rendered image of the pelvic floor to assess the position of the suburethral sling. Is it in place?
    a. Yes
    b. No
    c. Cannot tell from this image

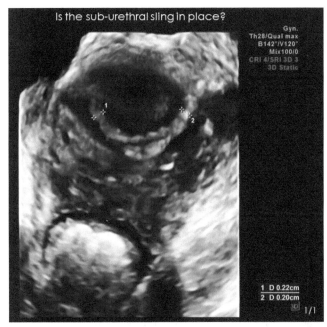

Fig. 221

CASE 104, FIGURES 222–224

22. Figs. 222–224 are those, using a 4–8 MHz EV transducer, of a 24-year-old female with deep pelvic aching. Fig. 222 is a transverse cut of the mid-uterus. Fig. 223 is a 3D volume set of the uterus with a transverse sweep plane. Note that all planes demonstrate a mottled uterine echo pattern. Fig. 224 is a sagittal cut through engorged lateral uterine vasculature. Based on the three images, what is the most likely diagnosis?
    a. Adenomyosis
    b. Leiomyomata
    c. Pelvic congestion
    d. Endometrial carcinoma
    e. Myometritis

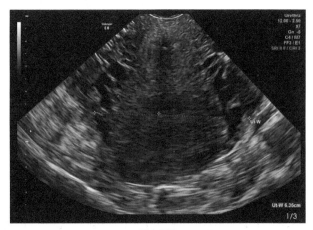

Fig. 222

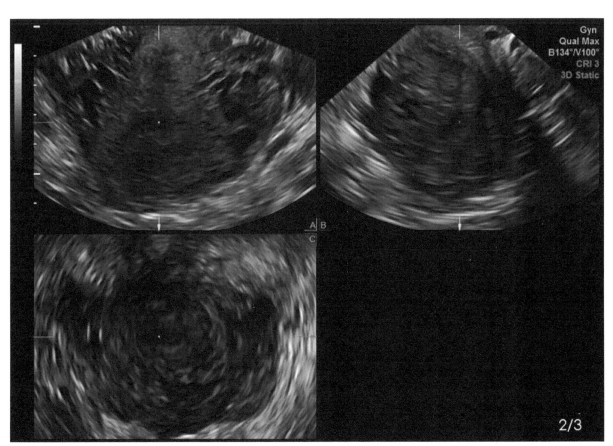

Fig. 223

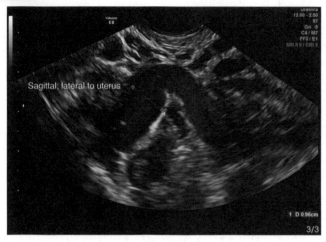

Fig. 224

CASE 105, FIGURE 225

23. Fig. 225 is a 3D volume set on a patient thought to have an enlarged uterus on clinical pelvic exam. Plane 1 is another ultrasound machine vendor's name for the A plane of a 3D volume set and is labeled on the screen slightly differently. Remember, the sweep plane is determined by the examiner. On what plane is the 3D volume sweep done?
    a. Sagittal
    b. Transverse
    c. Coronal

24. Identify the three numbered (3D) orthogonal planes.
    a. Plane 1 _____
    b. Plane 2 _____
    c. Plane 3 _____

25. Of the following, identify the uterine condition as seen by this volume set.
    a. Uterine didelphys
    b. Bicornuate uterus
    c. Septate uterus
    d. Arcuate uterus
    e. Unicornuate uterus

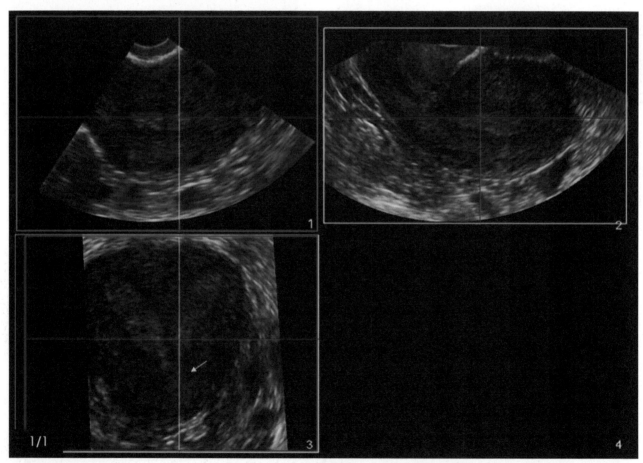

Fig. 225

CASE 106, FIGURE 226

26. Fig. 226 is a midsagittal image of the uterus following a sonohysterogram. Note the red arrow. What anatomic finding is suggested?
    a. At least one tube patency
    b. Bilateral tubular patency
    c. Bilaterally blocked tubes
    d. Intraperitoneal ascites

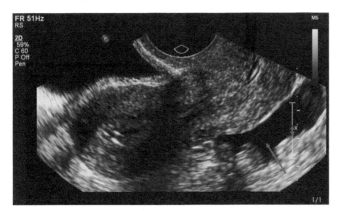

Fig. 226

CASE 107, FIGURE 227

27. Fig. 227 demonstrates two images of the uterus and bladder of a 76-year-old patient with complete procidentia. The top image is made with direct placement of the 5–9 MHz EV transducer on the externalized prolapsed pelvic structures. Transverse and sagittal planes on the prolapsed uterus and bladder are out of context and altered from typical relative location. Once the prolapse was reduced, the second image was taken, which demonstrates an EV view of the bulky enlarged bladder and a small uterus (gold arrow).

Imaging of these patients will rarely look the same due to the varied positions of the externalized anatomic structures. The patient subsequently underwent an elective colpocleisis. Look at the bladder contour on Fig. 227. Which of the following statements is not true?
    a. The bladder contour appears irregular and normal.
    b. The bladder contour appears bulky and abnormal.
    c. The bladder contour appears regular and abnormal.
    d. The bladder contour appears irregular and abnormal.

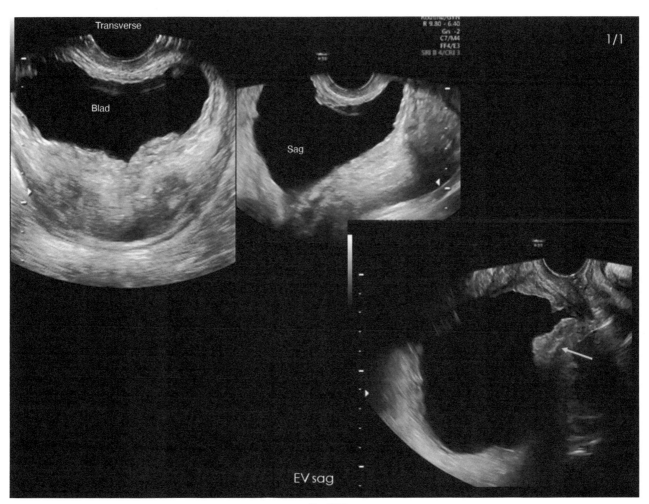

Fig. 227

CASE 108, FIGURES 228 AND 229

28. Figs. 228 and 229 are those of 28-year-old female who was diagnosed with severe pelvic congestion at her first pregnancy 17 months ago. Her last menstrual period was 5 days ago. She continues to experience pelvic pain and fullness. Which of the following is diagnostic criteria for her pain source?
    a. Profound peri-uterine dilated vessels
    b. Profound endometrial intracavitary hypervascularity
    c. Profound diffuse uterine vascularity
    d. Profound peripheral leiomyomata hypervascularity

29. Cumulative 3D hypervascularity is tricky because the 3D rendered image created from a 3D volume set is really an accumulation of multiple single images of a volume (Fig. 229) that one sees additively in the exam room; so, until the volume can be rotated, marked hypervascularity may be underappreciated. What is the most likely diagnosis for this finding?
    a. Endometritis
    b. Myometritis
    c. Leiomyomata
    d. Cervicitis
    e. Pelvic congestion

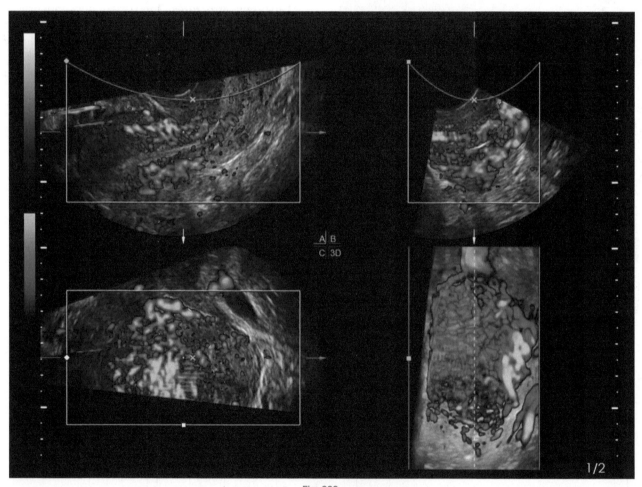

Fig. 228

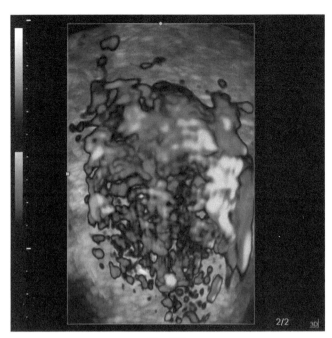

Fig. 229

CASE 109, FIGURES 230 AND 231

30. Fig. 230 is a transperineal axial cut at the midlevel of the internal anal sphincter (IAS) on a 51-year-old patient. The bolded *horizontal* calipers along the image left side are 1 cm. Fig. 231 is the 3D volume set of the anal sphincter complex on the same patient. Remember that the A plane is this ultrasound machine vendor's name for plane 1 of another vendor's 3D volume set and is labeled on the screen at the center of the four quadrants (white arrow).

a. Is the contour of the IAS circumferentially symmetric? _____
b. Is the IAS intact? _____
c. Is there elevation of the central mucosa? _____
d. Does the sagittal A plane (Fig. 231) demonstrate the disruption? _____
e. Does the C plane demonstrate that the center reference point (red arrows) is above the IAS? _____

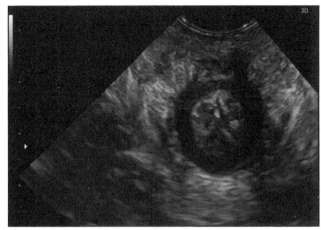

Fig. 230

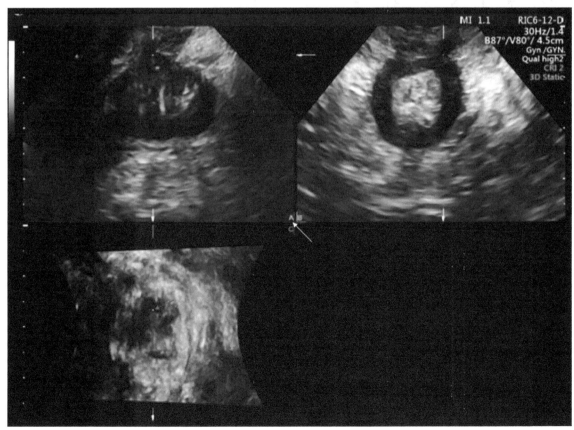

Fig. 231

CASE 110, FIGURE 232

31. The red arrows of Fig. 232 point to what structures at the midsagittal lower uterine segment/cervix image?
    a. Abnormal nabothian cysts
    b. Normal vaginal cysts
    c. Normal nabothian cysts
    d. Abnormal endometrial cysts

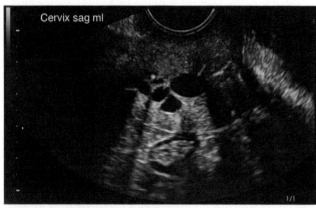

Fig. 232

CASE 111, FIGURES 233–238

32. Figs. 233–236 demonstrate EV 2D and 3D uterine images of a nulliparous 40-year-old patient referred for pelvic fullness and a clinically enlarged uterus, with no history of a previous imaging study. Based on this exam, she has a uterine volume of 829.28 cm³. What is the typical uterine volume? _____

33. There is clear evidence of an intrauterine mass, measuring 6 × 6 × 6 cm (Fig. 233; 3D volume set with the A plane sagittal, the B plane transverse, and the C plane coronal cuts of the mass). Which three of the following characteristics does it have?
    a. Poorly circumscribed borders
    b. Well-circumscribed borders
    c. Isoechoic relative to the myometrium
    d. Hypoechoic relative to the myometrium
    e. Hyperechoic relative to the myometrium
    f. Homogeneous echo pattern
    g. Heterogeneous echo pattern

34. Which of the following patterns of vascular flow do the Color Power Doppler images of the mass (Figs. 234–236) demonstrate?
    a. Diffuse intramass flow
    b. Focal peripheral flow around mass
    c. Diffuse peripheral around mass
    d. Focal intramass flow

35. Fig. 236 is the rendered image from the volume set. To what direction *on the patient* is the red arrow pointing?
    a. Left side
    b. Right side
    c. Superiorly
    d. Inferiorly

36. The patient returned 1 week later as seen on Figs. 237 and 238. How has the mass changed since the previous exam of 1 week ago relative to the following?
    a. Size (same, larger, smaller) _____
    b. Contour (regular, smooth, irregular, jagged) _____
    c. Shape (circular, trapezoidal, oblong, squared off) _____
    d. Echo pattern (same, homogeneous, less heterogeneous, more heterogeneous) _____
    e. Vascular pattern (same, increased peripheral vascularity, decreased peripheral vascularity, increased central vascularity, decreased central vascularity) _____

37. Which of the following is the most likely diagnosis?
    a. Leiomyosarcoma
    b. Endometrial carcinoma
    c. Leiomyoma, degenerating
    d. Leiomyoma, exophytic

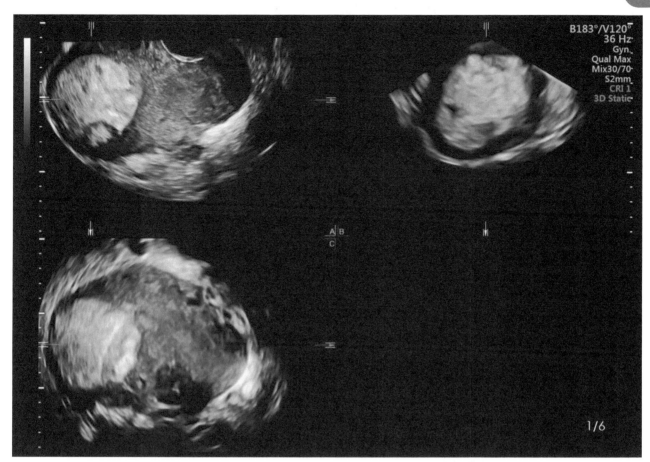

Fig. 233

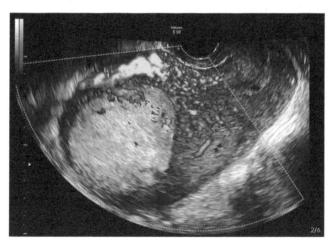

Fig. 234

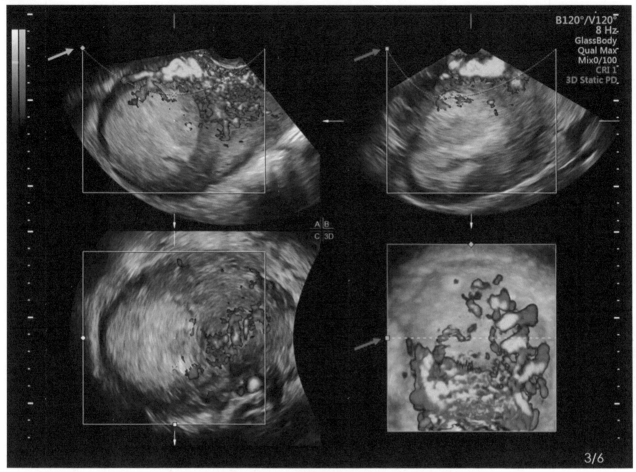

Fig. 235

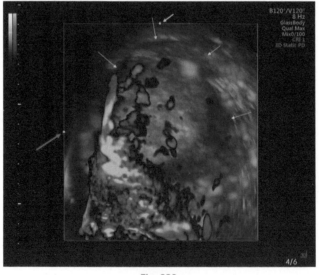

Fig. 236

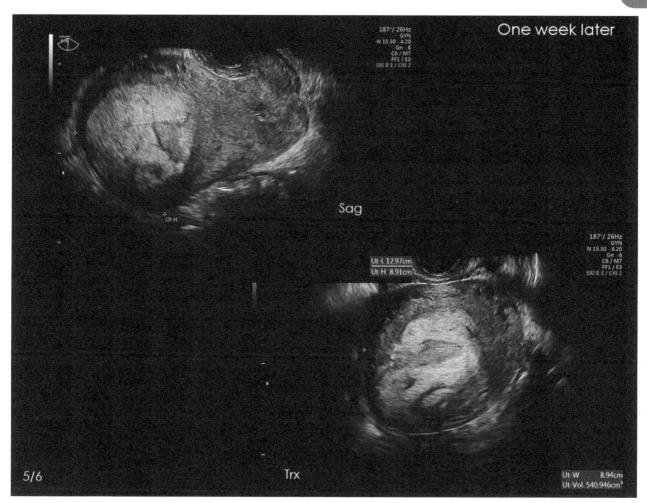

Fig. 237

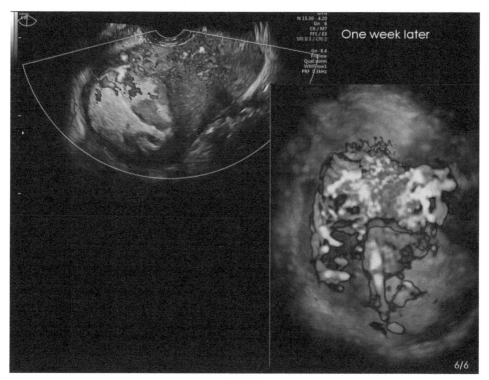

Fig. 238

Case Reviews 112–128

TOPIC 7, FIGURE 239

1. Fig. 239. Topic: Tomographic Ultrasound Imaging (TUI) of the Abnormal Transperineal Anal Sphincter Complex (ASC) 3D Volume Set

   When the ASC is abnormal, the use of TUI may illuminate the overall abnormal anatomic changes by demonstrating consistent proximal to distal cuts through the area in any plane. In this case, the axial cuts, made of 1-mm segments, demonstrate abnormal mid to distal changes of the internal anal sphincter and external anal sphincter integrity beginning at the mid central cut –3 to cut 3.

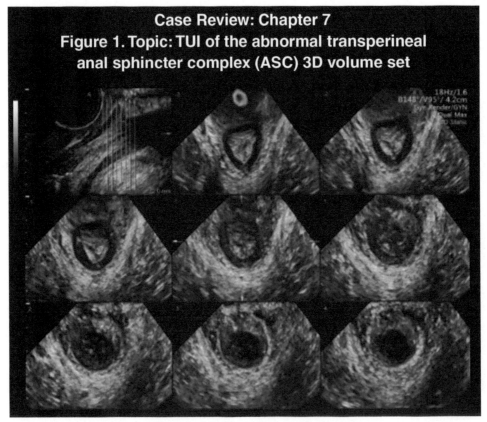

Fig. 239

CASE 112, FIGURE 240

2. Fig. 240 demonstrates two transperineal 3D rendered images of a normal suburethral sling, each with a different post-processed image type. Though the goal of surgery is to place the urethral sling posterior to the mid-urethral level, imaging may be utilized to determine at what level it is actually located; therefore, these imaging cases will generically call it "suburethral." The image on the left is a chroma-enhanced image and the one on the right is a tissue-enhanced image. Although the information is the same for each image, perception may be altered, and anatomy clarified with the type of post-processing at the time of the exam or later at the workstation. Instrumentation tools allow the examiner to manipulate the images on any axis, with any chroma type or any degree of individualized preference. Take the time to most optimally utilize the special functions on your ultrasound system.

The slight asymmetry of each side of the sling is within normal limits in appearance. Notice that the sling appears centrally positioned posterior to the urethra, although without the A plane of the 3D volume set, one cannot determine if it is located at the mid-urethra.

Answer the following questions.
a. Which appears crisper? _____
b. Which demonstrates visualization of the urethra better? _____
c. Which demonstrates visualization of the vagina better? _____
d. Which demonstrates the sling better? _____

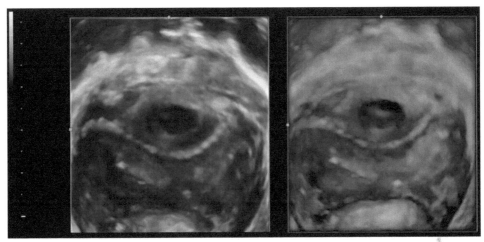

Fig. 240

CASE 113, FIGURES 241–243

3. Figs. 241 and 242 represent transperineal 3D volume set images using a 6–12 MHz endovaginal (EV) transducer of a 52-year-old patient who had unsuccessful placement of a urethral sling at an outside institution, which was ultimately "removed." In addition to her ongoing discomfort, she has returned to a urinary incontinence status.

Ideally, the mesh would be placed at the midlevel. Fig. 241 is a 3D volume set where the center reference point (CRP; gold arrows) is placed on which location below?
a. Proximal posterior urethral wall
b. Proximal anterior urethral wall
c. Mid anterior vaginal wall
d. Mid posterior vaginal wall
e. Distal posterior urethral wall
f. Distal anterior urethral wall

4. Fig. 241. With any standard pelvic floor 3D volume set, the anatomical cuts seen on the three orthogonal planes are relative to CRP placement, so it is operator dependent. Furthermore, with the line of reference brought from the top of the screen to the CRP and if residual mesh is present, it would be seen on the rendered image as a curvilinear suburethral structure and as an echogenic focus on the plane at the sagittal mid-urethral level and most optimally on the C plane. (The rendered image has been removed). Considering that the length of a urethra is approximately 4 cm, it is understandable that the mesh presence may not be appreciated at all even with a 1 cm error in CRP placement (see proximal, mid, and distal levels on the A plane at the blue, yellow, and red lines). Is there mesh seen at the midlevel? _____

5. The CRP (seen as the white, red, and light blue dots) on all three orthogonal planes on Fig. 241 was moved inferiorly on the volume set of Fig. 242

(gold arrows toward the top of the screen, which is inferior on the patient) and demonstrates how the diagnosis can be completely altered by changing where the CRP is placed. Remember, the ultrasound system will give you another place to see those intersecting center reference points with the partial arrows on the edges of each plane (pink arrows), no matter to where the CRP is moved. If residual mesh is present at this level, it would be seen. Is there mesh seen at this level? _____

6. At which location below is the CRP placed on Fig. 242?
   a. Proximal posterior urethral wall
   b. Proximal anterior urethral wall
   c. Mid posterior wall
   d. Mid anterior urethral wall
   e. Distal posterior urethral wall
   f. Proximal anterior urethra wall
   g. Proximal posterior urethral wall

The post-processed Fig. 243 is the C plane, now rotated upright on the Z-axis with the CRP (white dot; red arrow) seen *at* the residual mesh, extending along the mid to left lateral side of the proximal urethra (green arrows). Without visualization of a right mesh aspect (gold arrow), it was theoretically partially resected.

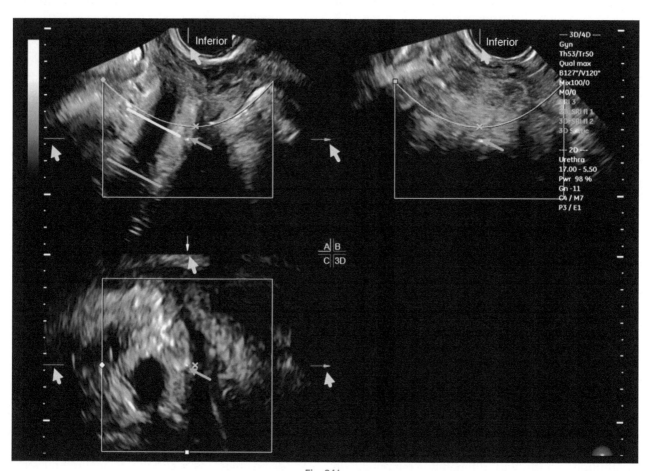

Fig. 241

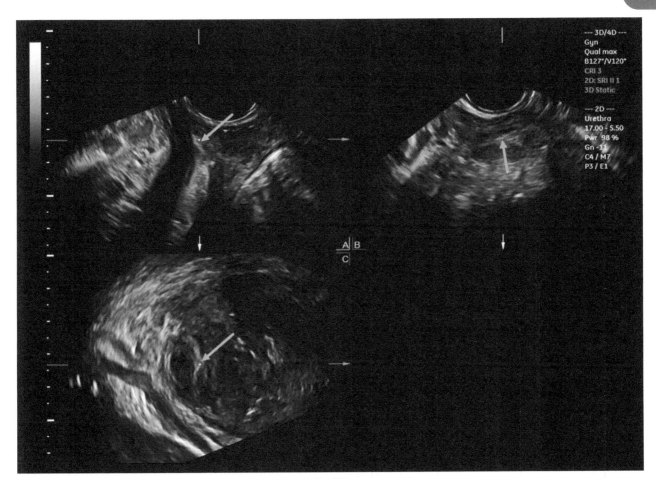

Fig. 242

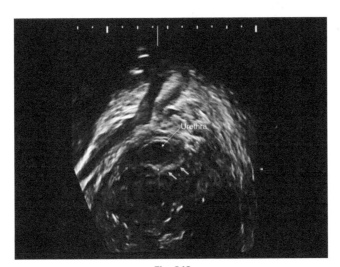

Fig. 243

CASE 114, FIGURES 244–246

7. Figs. 244–246 are those of a 45-year-old patient referred for a possible rectovaginal fistula using a 5–9 MHz EV transducer. Which one of the following image findings is *not* correct?
   a. The internal anal sphincter (IAS) is disrupted from 11–3 OC.
   b. There is no measurable IAS at 1 OC and 3 OC.
   c. There is elevation of the central mucosa toward the defect.
   d. There is isoechoic tracking noted extending from anterior 12 OC IAS to the patient's right.
8. Notice the gold arrows' distinct thin line appearance along the tracking on Fig. 246.
   Which is the correct diagnosis?
   a. IAS disruption with no evidence of a rectovaginal fistula
   b. IAS disruption with concomitant rectovaginal fistula

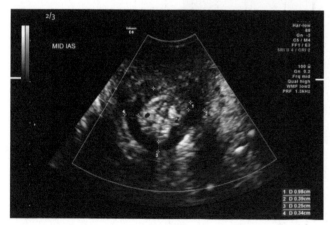

Fig. 244

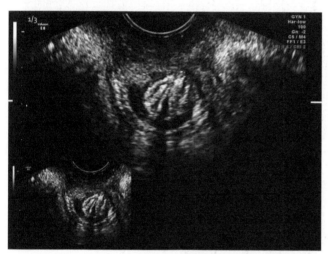

Fig. 245

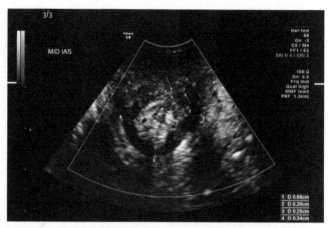

Fig. 246

CASE 115, FIGURE 247

9. Fig. 247 demonstrates a transperineal 3D volume set, using a 5–9 MHz EV transducer, of the pelvic floor. The A plane is a midsagittal image, the B plane is coronal, and the C plane is transverse of the pelvic floor structures. On what anatomical structure is the center reference point placed as seen on all three orthogonal cuts?
   a. Anterior vaginal wall
   b. Anterior rectal wall
   c. Mid-urethral mucosa
   d. Posterior vaginal/anterior rectal wall interface
   e. Posterior rectal wall
10. The 3D rendered image demonstrates a view of the pubovisceralis musculature from anterior (screen top) to posterior (screen bottom) on Fig. 247.
    a. Is the vaginal contour symmetric bilaterally? _____
    b. Is there any evidence of an avulsion? _____
    c. Is the pubovisceralis muscle complex symmetric bilaterally? _____

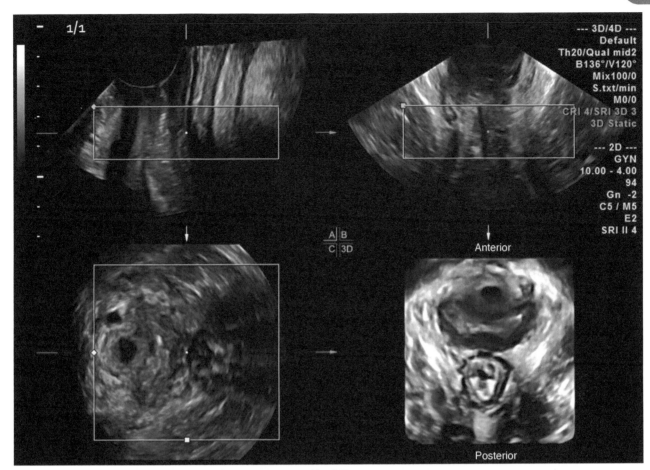

Fig. 247

CASE 116, FIGURE 248

11. Which of the images on Fig. 248 demonstrates an avulsion—A or B? _____

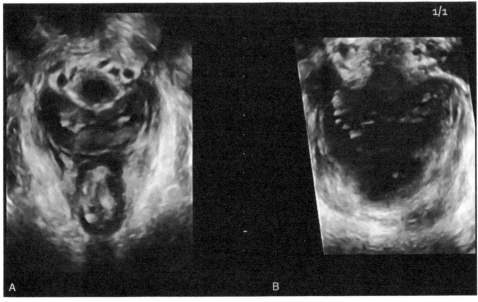

Fig. 248

CASE 117, FIGURE 249

12. Fig. 249 demonstrates a transperineal urethral image of a 55-year-old at rest and with cough. Which of the following is not true?
    a. The urethra kinks horizontally with cough.
    b. The urethral neck funnels with cough.
    c. There is a cystocele seen with cough.
    d. There is normal bladder appearance with cough.

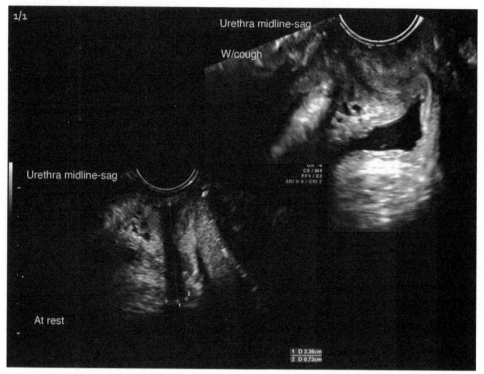

Fig. 249

CASE 118, FIGURE 250

13. From where to where (o'clock location) does Fig. 250 demonstrate a mid-internal anal sphincter disruption? _____
14. Is there elevation of the central mucosa? _____
15. Is there decreased, normal, or increased vascularity on the Color Power Doppler image of this anal sphincter complex area? _____

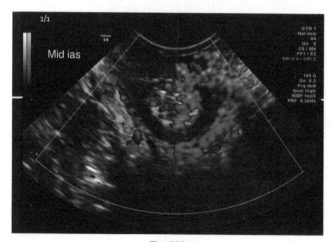

Fig. 250

CASE 119, FIGURES 251 AND 252

16. Figs. 251 and 252 demonstrate a transperineal 3D volume set and rendered 3D images using a 5–9 MHz EV transducer of the pelvic floor on a 59-year-old patient after a reported history of postoperative pain and continued incontinence following a suburethral sling procedure at an outside institution. "Removal" of mesh was performed, followed by worsening pain. The patient now presents to reassess the pelvic floor. Answer the following:
    a. The 3D acquisition A plane is a transperineal midsagittal cut. On what anatomical structure is the center reference point placed? _____
    b. At what level of the urethra is it located—proximal, mid, or distal? _____
    c. Fig. 252. On which side of the post-processed 3D rendered image is the remaining sling still present—the right, mid, or left? _____

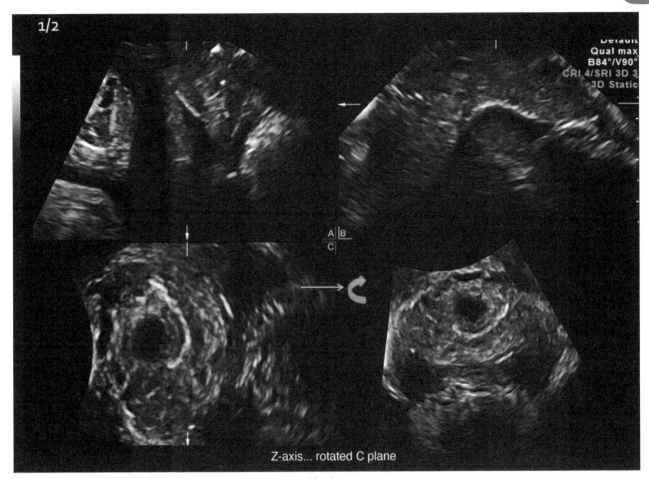

Fig. 251

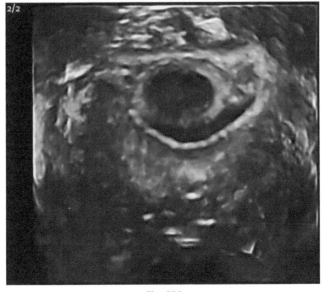

Fig. 252

CASE 120, FIGURES 253–260

17. Figs. 253–260 are images of a 27-year-old who had a pregnancy at age 17 that demonstrate the stark effect of early female circumcision. The patient had experienced an intrauterine fetal demise (IUFD) following a long labor, forceps delivery, and subsequent development of a rectal vaginal fistula. She underwent several surgeries in northeastern Africa to repair severe urinary incontinence, to no avail. This transperineal and endovaginal exam was performed using a 5–9 MHz EVtransducer to assess the anatomy.

Fig. 253 demonstrates a transperineal midline sagittal image of a very short urethra, measuring 1.04 cm (traced calipers) and a completely empty bladder.

Within minutes, her bladder began to spontaneously fill, as seen on Fig. 254. Adjacent to the bladder, a secondary hypoechoic area with a circumferentially thick hyperechoic wall became visualized (gold arrow). Relative to the bladder, in what location was this area located—posterior, anterior, superior, or inferior? _____

18. As the bladder was filling, Figs. 255–258 began to demonstrate a hypoechoic "tracking" on a 3D volume set between the two areas of fluid accumulation. With the use of the 3D volume set, the traced filling appeared to definitively originate from the bladder. With what appeared to be fluid freely tracking through to a secondary paravaginal location (gold arrow), her retroverted (RV) uterus began to be seen superiorly to the thick-walled, very short urethra (Fig. 257, gold arrow). With a 3D volume set, the center reference point was moved through the tracking, confirming it to be contiguous with the bladder (Fig. 258, rendered image).

Fig. 259. The filling bladder was soon elongated and markedly distorted, so much so that, as it could no longer sustain tone with the increasing quantity at only 14 cm³, it spontaneously released the urine onto the table. By placing the transducer intravaginally, as seen on Fig. 260, the RV uterus was clearly seen, with trace residual evidence of adjacent free fluid (gold arrow).

Based on your image assessment, which of the following is the likely tracking pathway? (From where to where is the tracking?)
a. Recto-vaginal fistula
b. Vesico-peritoneal fistula
c. Vesico-perineal fistula
d. Entero-vesico fistula

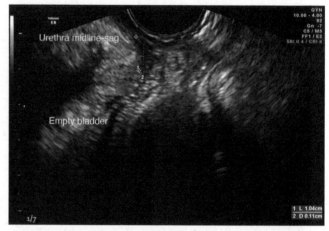

Fig. 253

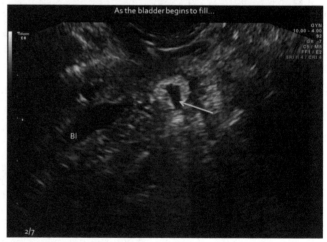

Fig. 254

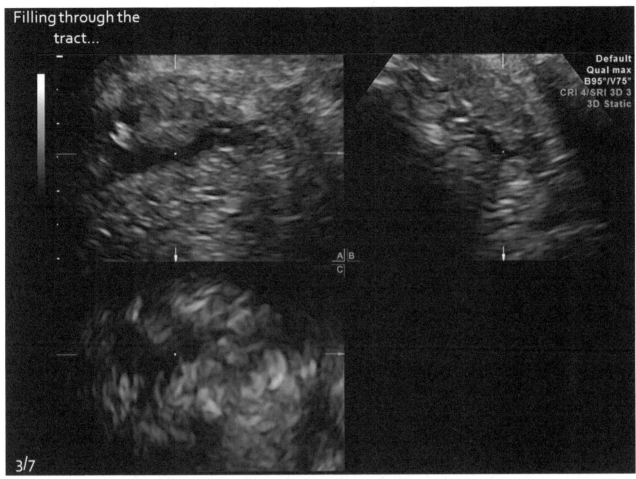

Fig. 255

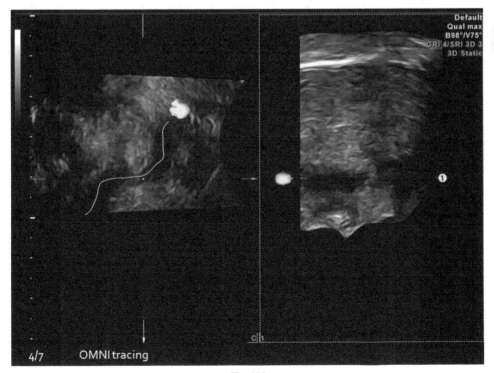

Fig. 256

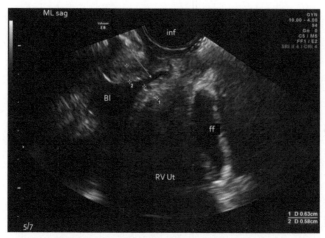

Fig. 257

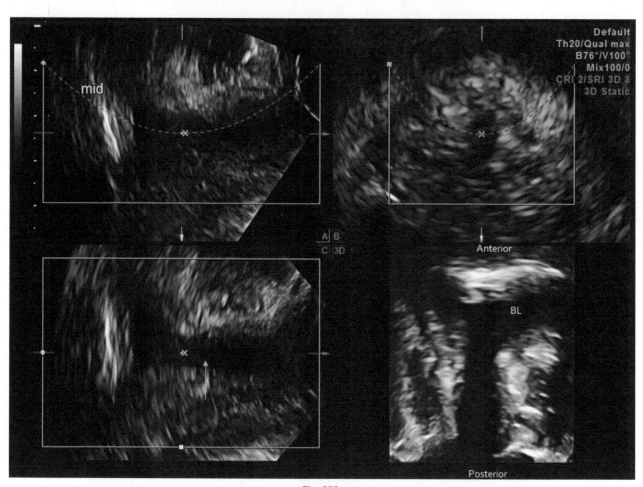

Fig. 258

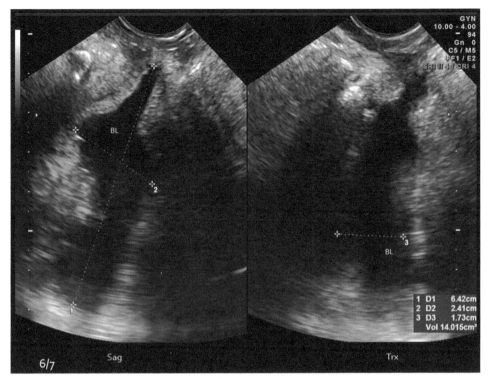

Fig. 259

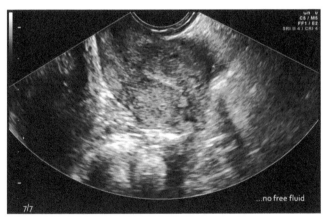

Fig. 260

CASE 121, FIGURE 261

19. Fig. 261. What is the length of a normal vagina? _____

20. Fig. 261 is a transperineal 2D midline sagittal image of the pelvic floor using 5–9 MHz EV transducer on a patient with clinically severe vaginal shortening. Because of its curved position, the length of the vagina was performed with a manual trace measurement caliper. What is the vaginal length on this exam? _____

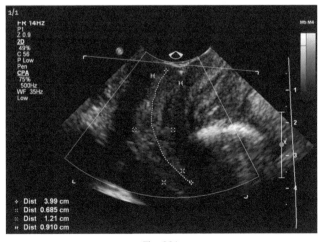

Fig. 261

CASE 122, FIGURES 262–267

21. Figs. 262–267 are multiple 2D and 3D transperineal images of the pelvic floor utilizing a 6–12 MHz EV transducer. The patient is a 53-year-old with a recent history of a suburethral sling placement and sacrocolpopexy, now presenting with severe vaginal/rectal pain. From the 2D midsagittal plane Fig. 262, identify the labeled *a–d* structures and directional *e–h* locations.

    a. _____

    b. _____

    c. _____

    d. _____

    e. _____

    f. _____

    g. _____

    h. _____

22. Fig. 263 is a 2D transperineal image of the urethra with maximum cough on the same patient. The suburethral sling is visualized (gold arrow) and does not move with the cough. Is it located at the proximal, mid, mid-distal, or distal urethra? _____

23. In Fig. 264, notice that on the 3D volume set, the proximal to mid-urethral mucosa is markedly widened (yellow arrow) *to* the location of the sling, beyond which it is significantly reduced in comparative anteroposterior diameter (white arrow). The center reference point (CRP) is placed just anterior to the sling. What are the three orthogonal planes at the CRP location relative to the urethra and relative to the body?

    a. Plane A _____

    b. Plane B _____

    c. Plane C _____

24. With the CRP moved to the sacrocolpopexy mesh on Fig. 265 (note white arrows pointing to colored CRP dots: white dot on A, red dot on B, and light blue dot on C planes), the rendered image now demonstrates the two mesh structures (blue arrows) at once. Relative to the directional green icons (diamond and square) at the edge of the four quadrants, what is the direction of the square (green arrows) of the rendered image on the patient?

    a. Right

    b. Left

    c. Inferior

    d. Superior

    e. Anterior

    f. Posterior

25. Fig. 266 demonstrates slightly manipulated rendered 3D rendered images with Y-axis rotation, allowing for complete imaging of the suburethral sling. If a calculation needs to be done post exam, calipers placed on a 3D rendered image reliably measure comparable distance between structures to 2D measurements. In this case, each line-to-line caliper is 1 cm and each line-to-dot is 0.5 cm. As an example, what is the distance from the suburethral sling to the sacrocolpopexy mesh? _____

26. Using ultrasound nomenclature, think about how you would report your exam findings.

    Fig. 267 exemplifies a report narrative for this case.

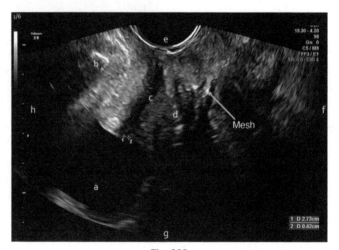

Fig. 262

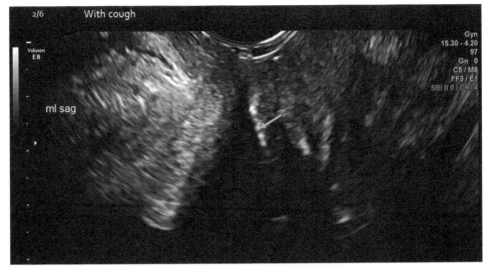

Fig. 263

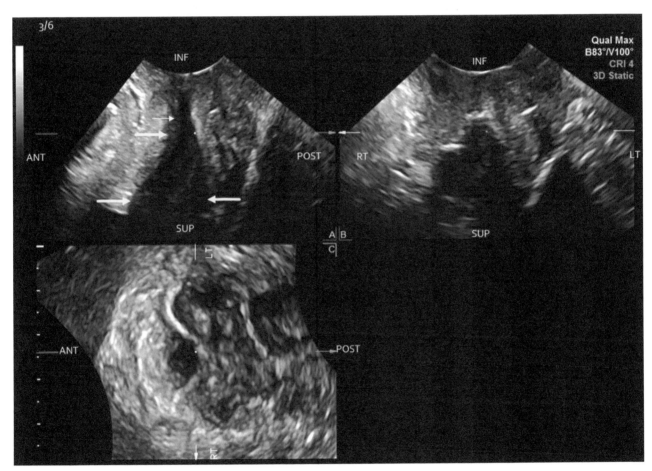

Fig. 264

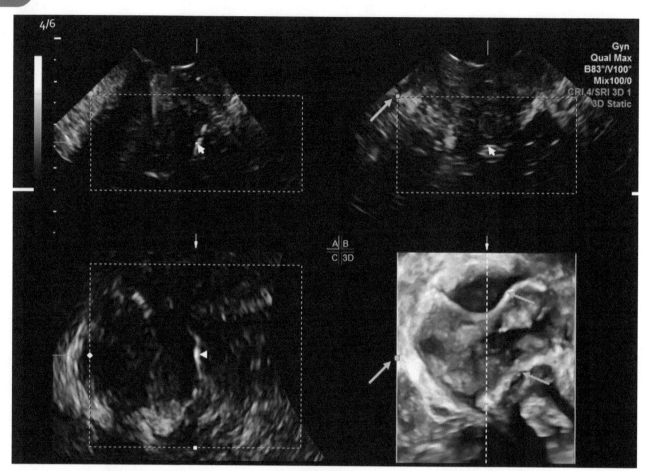

Fig. 265

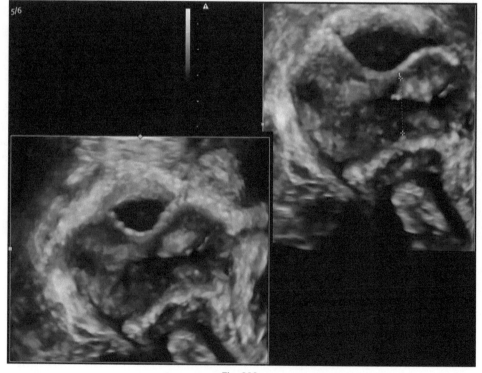

Fig. 266

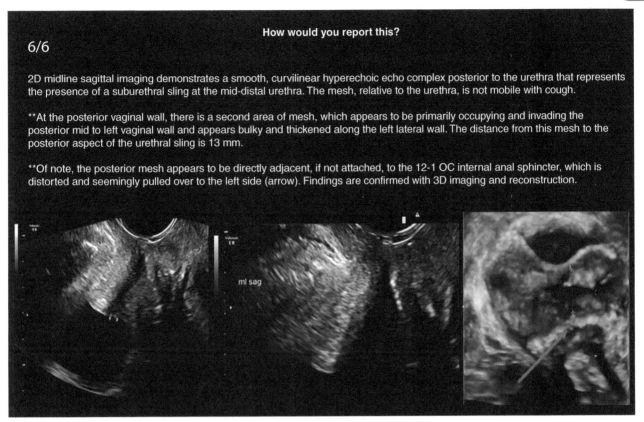

How would you report this?

6/6

2D midline sagittal imaging demonstrates a smooth, curvilinear hyperechoic echo complex posterior to the urethra that represents the presence of a suburethral sling at the mid-distal urethra. The mesh, relative to the urethra, is not mobile with cough.

**At the posterior vaginal wall, there is a second area of mesh, which appears to be primarily occupying and invading the posterior mid to left vaginal wall and appears bulky and thickened along the left lateral wall. The distance from this mesh to the posterior aspect of the urethral sling is 13 mm.

**Of note, the posterior mesh appears to be directly adjacent, if not attached, to the 12-1 OC internal anal sphincter, which is distorted and seemingly pulled over to the left side (arrow). Findings are confirmed with 3D imaging and reconstruction.

ml sag

Fig. 267

CASE 123, FIGURES 268–272

27. Figs. 268–272 demonstrate transperineal images of an autologous fascial sling using a 6–12 MHz EV transducer. The echo pattern of a fascial sling is not going to appear as distinct as a synthetic sling, nor will the structural shape be as definitive because the harvested fascial tissue is variable in shape and size. In this case, the size is small, about 2 × 2 cm, but appears deceivingly large on the small field of view high-frequency transperineal images. Fig. 268 demonstrates a 2D EV midsagittal image of the urethra with the isoechoic fascial sling seen at the mid suburethral location. The screen right image is post-processed to knock out the midlevel echoes and better demonstrate the fascial sling contour.

   With cough, as seen on Fig. 269, the contour, size, and location are better seen in addition to no movement of the fascial sling just posterior to the urethra. Using the calipers along the side of the image, with each line-to-line icon at 1 cm and each line-to-dot at 0.5 cm, measure the urethral length.

_____

28. Fig. 270 is a 3D volume set with the sweep plane a midsagittal cut and the center reference point (CRP) placed on the mid-urethra, just anterior to the fascial sling. The volume set is purposefully post-processed to high contrast to emphasize the fascial borders. Which of the three orthogonal planes best demonstrates the urethral wall/sling interface—A, B, or C? _____

29. As the CRP is moved to the fascial sling (Fig. 271) and the green line of reference is brought down to the CRP, the 3D rendered image (bottom right) is well defined as an irregularly shaped heterogeneous structure, definitively separate from the urethral wall. Fig. 272 demonstrates a 3D rendered and chroma-altered image of the marked comparatively asymmetric thickness of the fascial sling. From your perspective, how does the 3D image change the 2D gray scale appearance?
   a. Less quality with 3D
   b. The same quality with 3D
   c. Increased quality with 3D

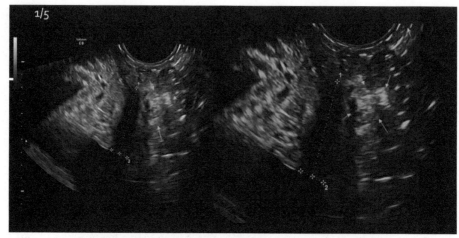

Fig. 268

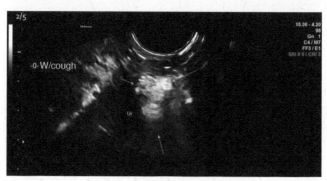

Fig. 269

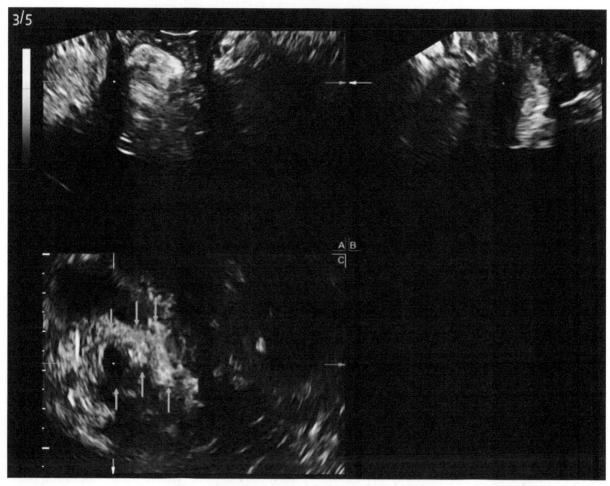

Fig. 270

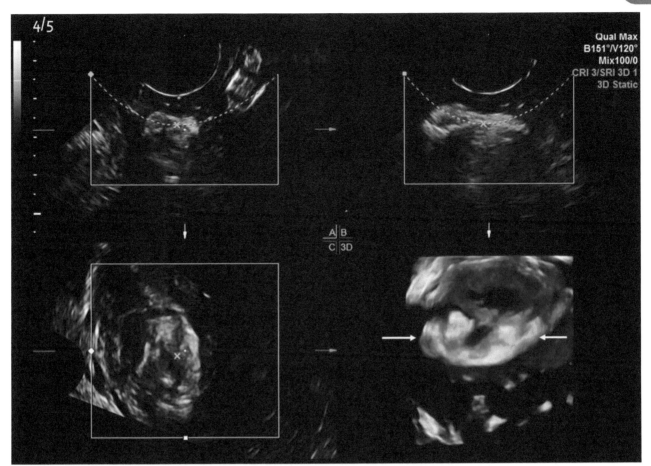

Fig. 271

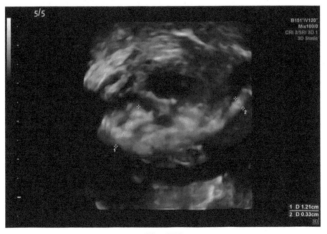

Fig. 272

CASE 124, FIGURE 273

30. Fig. 273 demonstrates a transperineal 3D volume set of the pelvic floor. The 3D rendered image has been removed and the C plane has been rotated on the Z-axis to bring the coronal plane of the pelvic floor upright, which may appear more intuitive to the examiner, especially the pubovisceralis muscle complex.

a. Where is the center reference point placed? _____

b. Is the bladder empty or full? _____

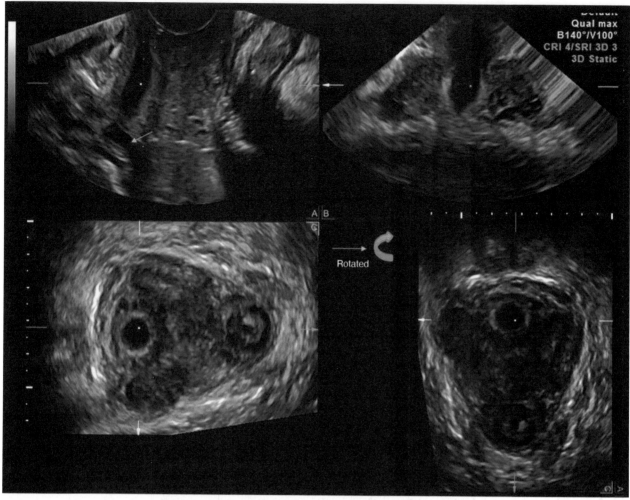

Fig. 273

CASE 125, FIGURE 274

31. Fig. 274 demonstrates two transperineal axial cuts of the IAS using a 5–9 MHz endovaginal transducer on two separate patients. The left image demonstrates an anteroposterior (AP) diameter of the hypoechoic IAS measuring a typical 2.5 mm, which appears symmetric at the 12, 3, 6, and 9 OC positions. The right image demonstrates a symmetric more hyperechoic IAS appearance, with the AP diameters at the 12, 3, 6, and 9 OC positions all measuring 5.5–6 mm. What is the most likely mechanism for this difference?

a. Stool in the rectum
b. Disruption distal to the proximal-level IAS
c. Disruption of the IAS from 5–7 OC
d. Compensatory IAS hypertrophy from external anal sphincter disruption

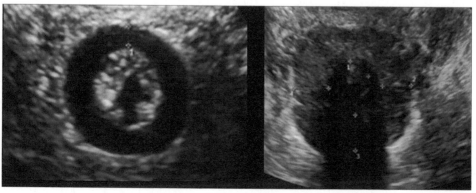

Fig. 274

CASE 126, FIGURE 275

32. Fig. 275 is a 2D transperineal axial cut of the mid-IAS using a 5–9 MHz endovaginal transducer. Is the IAS intact? _____

33. What does the Color Power Doppler indicate on Fig. 275? _____

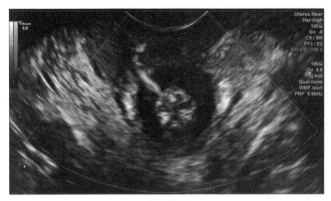

Fig. 275

CASE 127, FIGURES 276 AND 277

34. Figs. 276 and 277 demonstrate a 2D and a 3D volume set of a 63-year-old patient who is 6 weeks s/p Burch procedure performed at an outside institution, now presenting with persistent dysuria and pelvic pain. Urinary tract injury is evident on both 2D and 3D as a hyperechoic curvilinear structure extending across one side of the bladder to the other side, thought to represent a residual surgical stitch.

The 3D orthogonal planes demonstrate how a stitch "coming at you" on a 2D image may not be appreciated until the 3D rendered image is made.

"Looking in" from the side on the B plane at the volume, the green line of reference demonstrates the 3D rendered image all the way across the bladder. If the examiner was only performing a 2D exam of this bladder and saw the single echogenic focus within the full bladder, how could the 2D transducer be manipulated to see if the focus can be elongated? _____

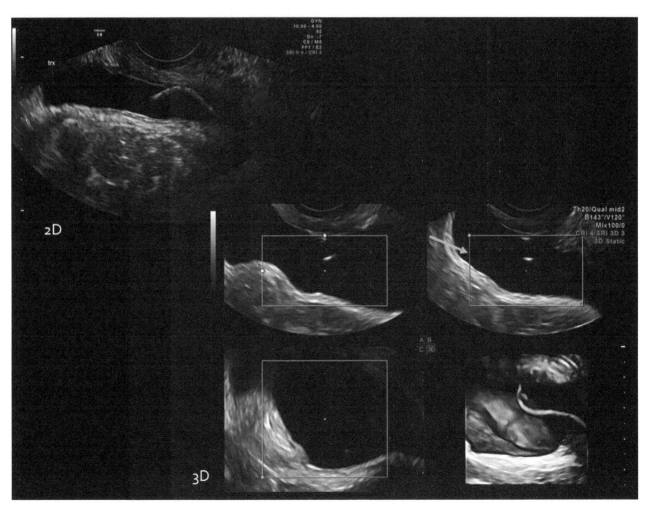

Fig. 276

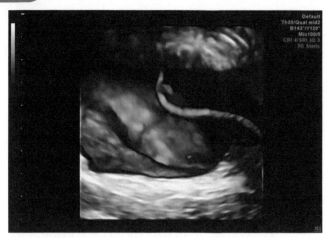

Fig. 277

CASE 128, FIGURE 278

35. Fig. 278 demonstrates transperineal axial images using a 5–9 MHz EV transducer of the mid-ASC on a 47-year-old patient suspected of having a rectovaginal fistula. The transducer is placed perpendicular to the table at the distal posterior vaginal wall; therefore, the axial cuts through the internal anal sphincter can be minimally angled from superiorly to inferiorly to find the level of abnormality on real time. The unusual appearance at the posterior vaginal wall/sphincter interface of a hyperechoic take off (blue arrow) and tracking (gold arrow) is noticeably "flickering" in real time. Which of the following descriptions best describes the abnormal finding?
   a. There is a hyperechoic curvilinear area thought to represent air extending anteriorly toward the transducer from the mid-ASC and extending to the patient's left, the finding c/w a rectovaginal fistula.
   b. There is a hyperechoic curvilinear area thought to represent air extending anteriorly toward the transducer from the right ASC and extending to the patient's left, the finding c/w a rectovaginal fistula.
   c. There is a hyperechoic curvilinear area thought to represent air extending anteriorly toward the transducer from the left ASC and extending to the patient's left, the finding c/w a rectovaginal fistula.
   d. There is a hyperechoic curvilinear area thought to represent air extending anteriorly toward the transducer from the mid-sphincter and extending to the patient's right, the finding c/w a rectovaginal fistula.

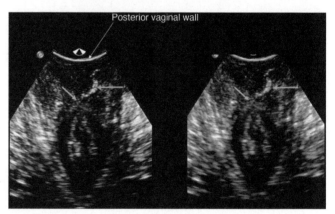

Posterior vaginal wall

Fig. 278

Case Reviews 129–150

TOPIC 8, FIGURE 279

1. Fig. 279. Topic: "Read" Zoom Versus "Write" Zoom.
   Magnifying an ultrasound image is commonly done by the examiner; however, making an image appear bigger by merely turning the zoom knob will only magnify each pixel ("read" zoom). As the image gets bigger, the frame rate (FR) or number of images per second will not be changed, and resolution of the image will depreciate as it is increased because all it does is make bigger pixels. If the examiner presses the high-resolution zoom knob, a box will come onto the screen, which can be changed (narrowed, lengthened, etc.) in size by the examiner in order to reacquire the acoustic lines at the area of interest within the box (it will "rewrite" the zoom). Doing this increases the FR and results in a zoomed image with higher resolution. The FR is seen on all images (yellow arrows) and can be seen to be the same at 50 Hz for the original and the read zoomed images, but at 95 Hz for the write zoomed image with improved resolution. Do not confuse the "frame rate" with the transducer "frequency."

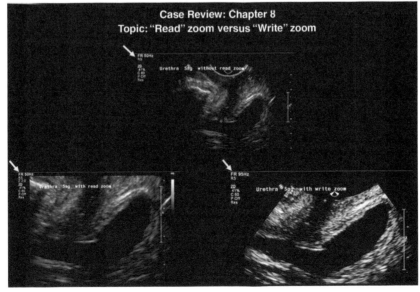

Fig. 279

CASE 129, FIGURE 280

2. Fig. 280 demonstrates 2D transverse and sagittal images of the right ovary, using a 4–8 MHz endovaginal (EV) transducer, on a 44-year-old multiparous patient referred for clinical adnexal fullness. The ultrasound assessment of the left ovary is normal and is not presented.

Measurements can be made post exam. Each line to dot or dot to line along the side of the image measures 0.5 cm. Which of the following is the correct abnormal right ovarian size based on the calipers along the side of the images?
   a. 20 × 12 × 10.4 cm
   b. 10 × 6 × 5.2 cm

3. Fig. 280. Which of the following best describes the ovarian mass echo pattern?
   a. Complex primarily cystic in appearance with multiple clusters of papillations around a single vertical septum
   b. Complex primarily solid in appearance with diffuse hypoechoic intraovarian mural wall nodules
   c. Anechoic in echo pattern with multiple, diffuse, round hyperechoic sub-lesions
   d. Heterogeneous with a complex primarily cystic appearance

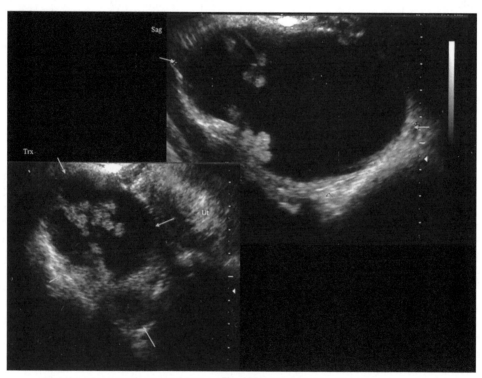

Fig. 280

CASE 130, FIGURE 281

4. Fig. 281 demonstrates images of a 32-year-old multiparous patient who presents with nonspecific but constant pelvic pain and dyspareunia. Both the ovaries are well visualized and appear within normal limits and are not presented. The top left image is a 2D EV midline sagittal image using a 5–9 MHz EV transducer and the bottom right is a post-processed transverse mid-uterus image to knock out midlevel echoes (to enhance contrast). Note that the uterus appears bulky in global appearance. The bottom left image demonstrates the Color Power Doppler vascular pattern. Based on these images, answer the following questions with Yes or No.
   a. The endometrium appears trilaminar in echo pattern. _____

   b. The uterus is diffusely homogeneous. _____
   c. The endometrial/myometrial interface appears indistinct. _____
   d. The myometrium contains diffuse small hypoechoic lesions. _____
   e. Normal nabothian cysts are present. _____

5. The sonographic findings are consistent with which two of the following?
   a. Adenomyosis
   b. Leiomyomata
   c. Uterine sarcoma
   d. Endometrial carcinoma

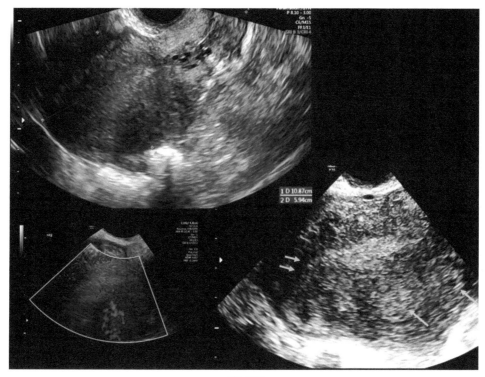

Fig. 281

CASE 131, FIGURES 282–284

6. Figs. 282–284 are images, using a 5–9 MHz 3D EV transducer, of a 50-year-old patient with a suspected right-sided pelvic mass found on clinical exam. The ultrasound assessment of the left ovary is normal and is not presented. The right adnexa appears as a complex primarily cystic appearing mass with an irregularly shaped hyperechoic subcomponent, measuring 1.67 × 2.85 × 2.15 cm, seen as a large mural nodule at the superior aspect of the mass (calipers). A septum is noted, extending vertically with an irregular varied thickness and a hyperechoic pattern. From the 3D volume set of the right ovary, approximate the adnexal mass dimensions. _____

7. Fig. 283 demonstrates the Color Power Doppler vascular flow pattern of the mass. The 2D image of Color Power Doppler (screen left) only demonstrates a single cut of the entire vascularity within or around a mass; therefore, the overall 3D rendered image (screen right) enhances the overall suspicion of an abnormal intramass component with visualization of diffuse markedly increased blood flow.

When there is questionable intramass hypervascularity, the examiner should turn down the pulse repetition frequency (PRF) to maximize the flow pattern. If the flow becomes "blushed" in appearance such that artifactual colors pixelate the entire color box, the PRF has been set too low. When this threshold is reached, the PRF can be incrementally increased to where the blush goes away, leaving the *real* minimal flow pattern, as seen on the 2D Color Power Doppler images.

Once increased vascularity is established, it is important to analyze vessels with Doppler spectral velocity waveform analysis as exemplified in Fig. 284. Velocities are presented on the screen when any quantitative Doppler spectral measurements are done. Which Doppler velocity index is the most reliable to evaluate ovarian flow pattern in the presence of hypervascularity—the peak systolic velocity (PSV), the end-diastolic velocity (EDV), or the resistive (RI) index? _____

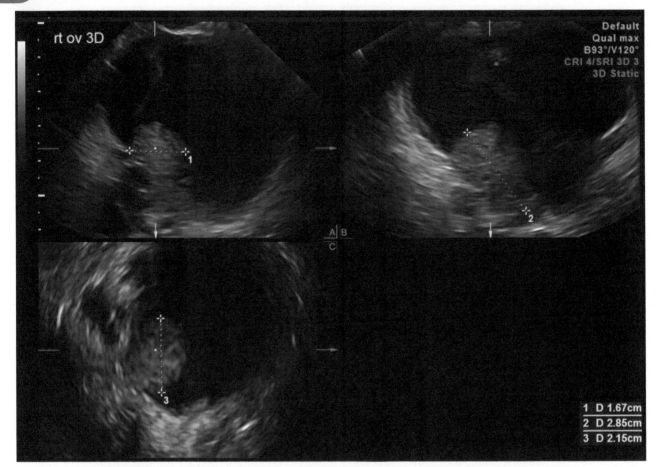

Fig. 282

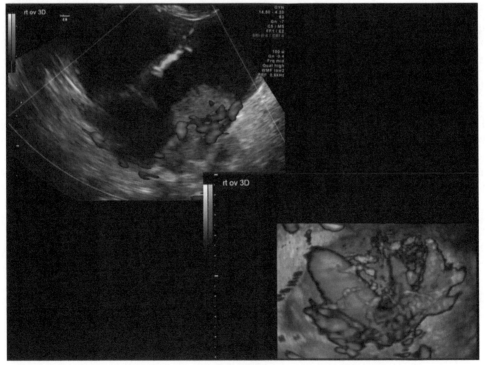

Fig. 283

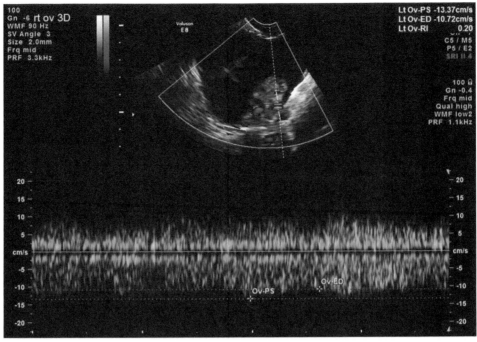

Fig. 284

CASE 132, FIGURE 285

8. Fig. 285 is a single 2D transperineal image of the internal anal sphincter (IAS) using a 6–12 MHz EV transducer. Answer the following questions.
   a. Are the anteroposterior dimensions of all four quadrants of the IAS symmetric? _____
   b. Is there a disruption of the IAS? _____
   c. Is there elevation of the central mucosa? _____
   d. At what level of the anal sphincter complex is this image made? _____

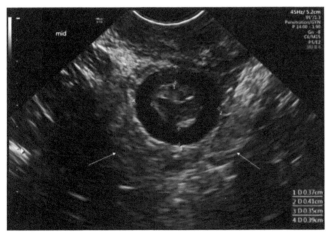

Fig. 285

CASE 133, FIGURE 286

9. Fig. 286 demonstrates the vaginal cuff using a 6–12 MHz EV transducer on a 36-year-old patient who is status post (s/p) transvaginal hysterectomy with a history of endometriosis and postoperative pain and dyspareunia. The screen top image demonstrates the most anterior vaginal cuff in a transverse plane. Note that the cuff is smooth in contour and homogeneous in echo pattern (gold arrows).

   Is the curvilinear cuff hyperechoic, isoechoic, or hypoechoic relative to the adjacent bladder wall?
   a. Hyperechoic
   b. Isoechoic
   c. Hypoechoic

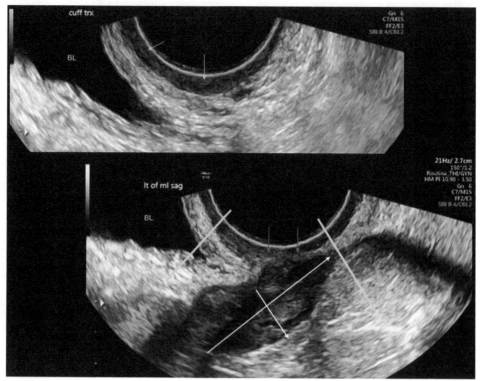

Fig. 286

CASE 134, FIGURES 287–291

10. Figs. 287–291 demonstrate transabdominal 2D pelvic and 3D rendered images of a patient with a living 13-week intrauterine pregnancy (IUP) using transabdominal 1–5 MHz and 2–6 MHz 3D transabdominal transducers. The left adnexa demonstrates a large, well-circumscribed, complex, primarily solid-appearing mass, measuring 13.5 × 9.19 × 12.06 cm, directly adjacent to the left aspect of the uterus with abundant vascularity noted (Fig. 287).
    a. Is the mass contiguous to or adjacent and separate from the uterus (Fig. 288)? _____
    b. Is the echogenicity of the mass hypoechoic, isoechoic, or hyperechoic as compared to the uterus? _____

11. With any pelvic mass, it is crucial to demonstrate the individual ovaries as separate or part of the mass. See Figs. 289 and 290. Does either ovary appear as part of the mass? Answer Yes or No.
    a. Left _____
    b. Right _____

12. Fig. 291 demonstrates a 3D rendered image of the IUP and adjacent mass and helps to demonstrate the relative size of the mass to the current size of the IUP. What is the volume of the mass? _____

13. Based upon the assessment considerations above, which of the following is the most likely diagnosis for this mass?
    a. Submucosal leiomyoma
    b. Exophytic subserosal leiomyoma
    c. Subserosal leiomyoma
    d. Pedunculated leiomyoma

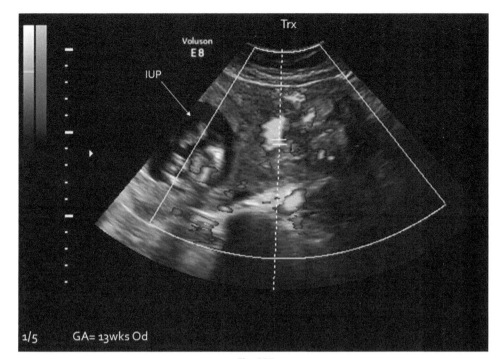

Fig. 287

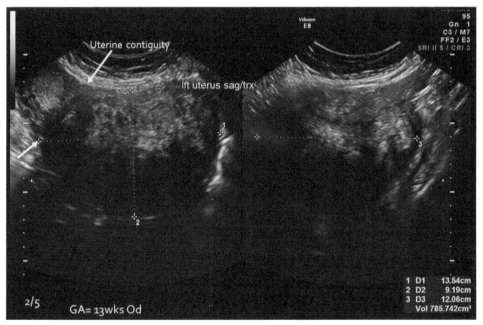

Fig. 288

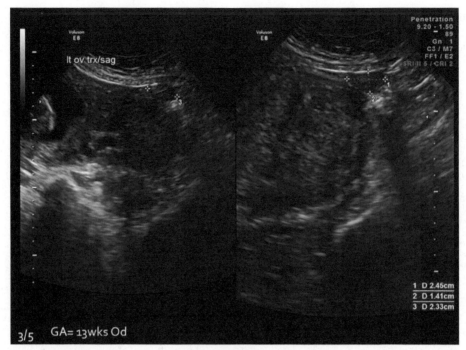

Fig. 289

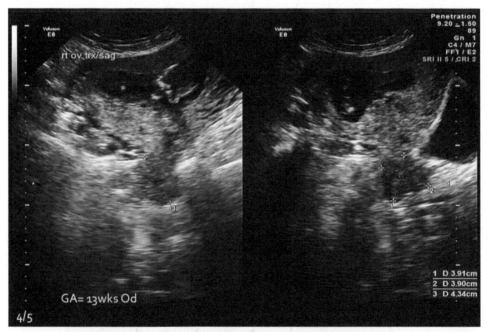

Fig. 290

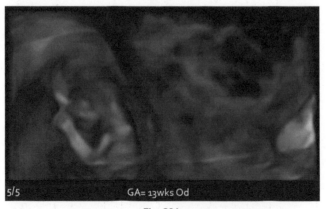

Fig. 291

CASE 135, FIGURE 292

14. Fig. 292 is labeled as a transverse image of the cervix (arrow) using a 4–8 MHz EV transducer. The entire cervical cut displays diffuse hypoechoic oval-shaped structures ranging in size from 2–20 mm, consistent with the presence of diffuse nabothian cysts. Does the number and size of the nabothian cysts raise concern for the provider? _____

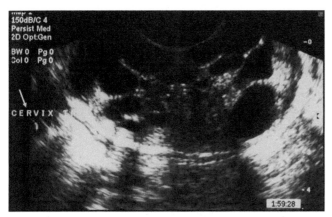

Fig. 292

CASE 136, FIGURE 293

15. Fig. 293 is an incidental finding at a midsagittal image of the lower uterine segment/cervical interface using a 5–9 MHz EV transducer when performing an exam for abnormal uterine bleeding. Does the image display Doppler Color Flow, Color Power Doppler, or a Doppler spectral waveform? _____

16. To what are the arrows pointing?
    a. Compression of the endometrium/ cervical interface by anterior myoma
    b. Elevated endometrium at cesarean scar
    c. Endometrial polyp
    d. Compression of the endometrium/cervical interface by posterior myoma

17. What is the distance from the most anterior aspect of the elevated interface to the anterior uterine wall?
    a. 1 mm
    b. 2 mm
    c. 3 mm
    d. 4 mm
    e. 5 mm

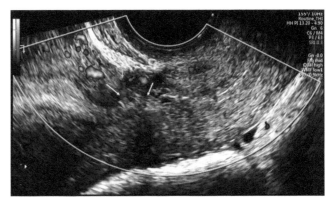

Fig. 293

CASE 137, FIGURE 294

18. Fig. 294 demonstrates two C plane transperineal images of a transobturator tape (TOT) taken out of context of two 3D volume sets using a 6–12 MHz EV transducer. With the swept volume available, the anatomy can be manipulated to rotate toward the lateral aspect of each mesh component.

    Which side of the patient is the mesh of image A? Right or Left? _____

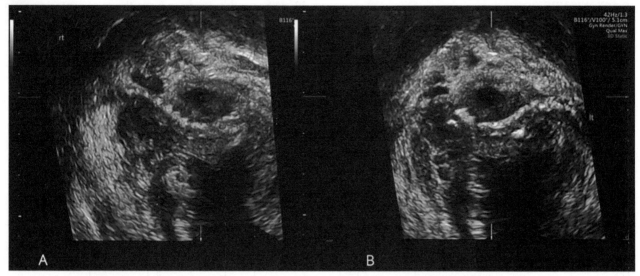

Fig. 294

CASE 138, FIGURES 295–297

19. Figs. 295–297 demonstrate an adnexal mass that was an incidental finding using a 5–9 MHz 3D EV transducer of a 46-year-old patient who was being examined for clinical pelvic fullness. Both the ovaries appear within normal limits and are not presented. Fig. 295 is a 2D image of a left adnexal multilocular appearing lesion located adjacent to the left ovary. By turning the transducer 90 degrees from the initial 2D image, this structure appears as a serpiginous structure folded over itself. (Fig. 296). With a 3D volume sweep of this plane, a 3D OMNI trace through the path of the tortuous anechoic structure (Fig. 297) was done ("stretched out"). This can only happen if the folds are contiguous, as is the appearance here. When stretched out, a true measurement can be made of the length (screen right). If it is NOT contiguous, it would indicate that the lesion is more than one structure. What is the most likely diagnosis for this adnexal mass?

a. Abnormal loop of small bowel
b. Dilated fallopian tube
c. Multiple paraovarian cysts
d. Dilated peripheral uterine hypervascularity

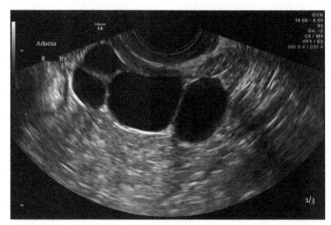

Fig. 295

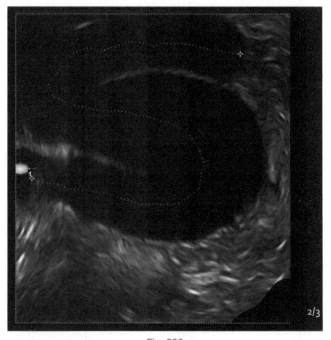

Fig. 296

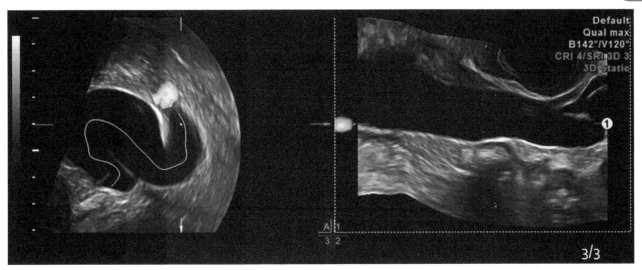

Fig. 297

CASE 139, FIGURES 298–301

20. Fig. 298–301 are those, using a 4–8 MHz EV transducer, of a 33-year-old patient who presented to the emergency room with acute left lower quadrant pain. Her last menstrual period was 15 days ago. Fig. 298 is a mid-uterus transverse image. The right ovary appears normal and is not presented. To what are the gold arrows pointing? _____

21. Figs. 299 and 300 are transverse cuts through the left ovary, 90 degrees to where the gold star is seen on the sagittal cut on Fig. 301. The ovary measures $4.2 \times 4.97 \times 5.2$ cm. Given its complex appearance, detailed reporting of the left ovary is important. Which of the following is the most optimal description of the left ovary?

a. The left ovary is comprised of an oval-shaped anechoic lesion measuring 2.59×1.65 cm adjacent to a smooth-walled hyperechoic mass measuring 3×4.5 cm.

b. The left ovary is comprised of bilobular masses with an anechoic anterior segment measuring 2.59×1.65 cm adjacent to a homogeneous posterior segment measuring 3×4.5 cm.

c. The left ovary is comprised of bilobular masses with an anechoic anterior segment measuring 2.59×1.65 cm adjacent to a heterogeneous posterior segment measuring 3×4.5 cm.

d. The left ovary is comprised of an oval-shaped heterogeneous lesion measuring 2.59×1.65 cm adjacent to a smooth-walled hyperechoic mass measuring 3×4.5 cm.

22. Which of the following is *not* a sonographic differential diagnosis for the above findings?

a. Hemorrhagic corpus luteum
b. Bilobular follicular cysts
c. Left ovarian neoplasm
d. Endometrioma

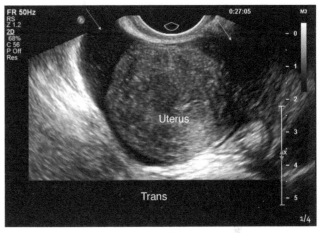

Fig. 298

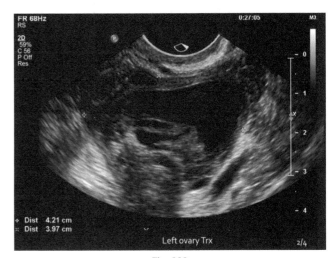

Fig. 299

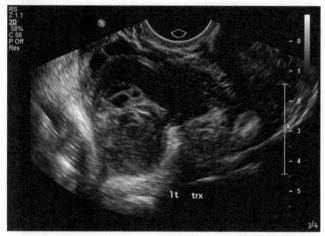

Fig. 300

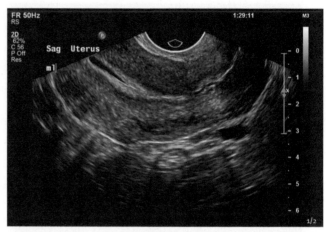

Fig. 302

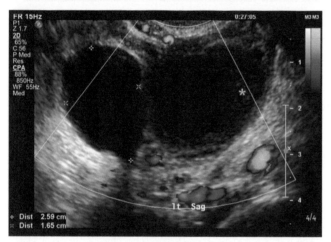

Fig. 301

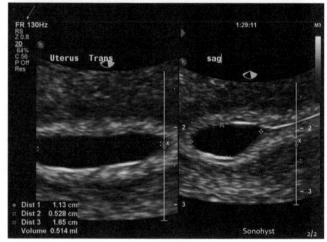

Fig. 303

CASE 140, FIGURES 302 AND 303

23. Fig. 302 demonstrates a midsagittal image of the uterus using a 4–8 MHz EV transducer at the end of a sonohysterogram during which time 5 cc of normal saline had been infused into the endometrial cavity. Fig. 303 demonstrates write zoomed images of the cavity in sagittal and transverse cuts. Which **two** of the following options indicate that Fig. 303 images were "write" zoomed versus "read" zoomed?
   a. The image resolution is higher on Fig. 303 versus Fig. 302.
   b. The image resolution is higher on Fig. 302 versus Fig. 303.
   c. The frame rate is higher on Fig. 302 versus Fig. 303.
   d. The frame rate is higher on Fig. 303 versus Fig. 302.

CASE 141, FIGURE 304

24. Fig. 304 is a midsagittal image of the anteverted uterus of a 38-year-old patient using a 5–9 MHz EV transducer. In what phase of the endometrial cycle does this image suggest?
   a. Early proliferative
   b. Late proliferative
   c. Mid-cycle
   d. Secretory

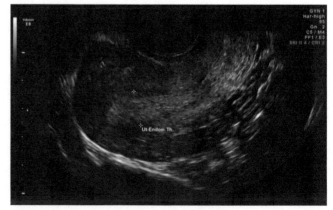

Fig. 304

CASE 142, FIGURES 305–308

25. Figs. 305–308 are 2D images of a 41-year-old patient using a 4–8 MHz EV transducer to evaluate the right ovary, which was thought to appear abnormal on another ultrasound exam 3 weeks ago. The left ovary appeared normal on both exams and is not demonstrated. Note that the right ovary measures normal at 3.3 × 2.5 × 2.47 cm.

Though the ovarian volume is within normal limits, there is a well-circumscribed heterogeneous central subcomponent seen on both sagittal and transverse planes measuring 2.47 × 2.10 cm. Within the subsegment, there are multiple anechoic, oval-shaped structures measuring up to 13 mm as seen in Fig. 307 (gold arrows). Additionally, there appears to be the presence of several strand-like linear structures (red arrows, Fig. 307) within the subcomponent, and Doppler spectral waveform of the vascularity elicits a resistive index (RI) of 0.38 (Fig. 308).

Which of the following is the *least* likely etiology for these findings?
a. Simple corpus luteum
b. Ovarian neoplasm
c. Follicular cysts
d. Hemorrhagic corpus luteum
e. Multiple follicles

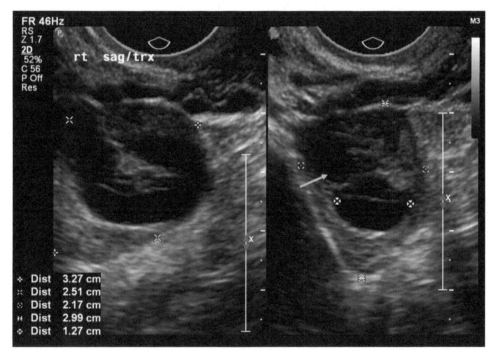

Fig. 305

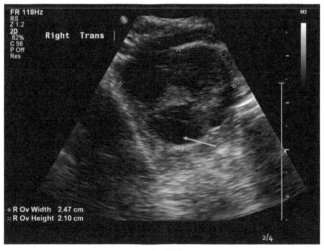

Fig. 306

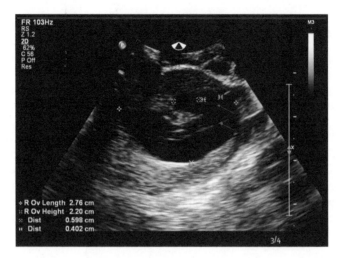

Fig. 307

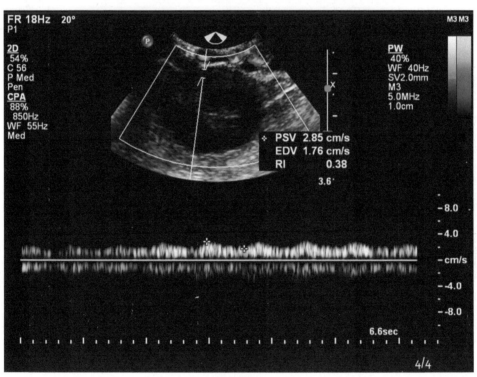

Fig. 308

CASE 143, FIGURE 309

26. Fig. 309 is a transperineal pelvic floor 3D volume set on a patient with anal incontinence. Based on the C plane and rendered images, is there an evidence of an avulsion injury? _____

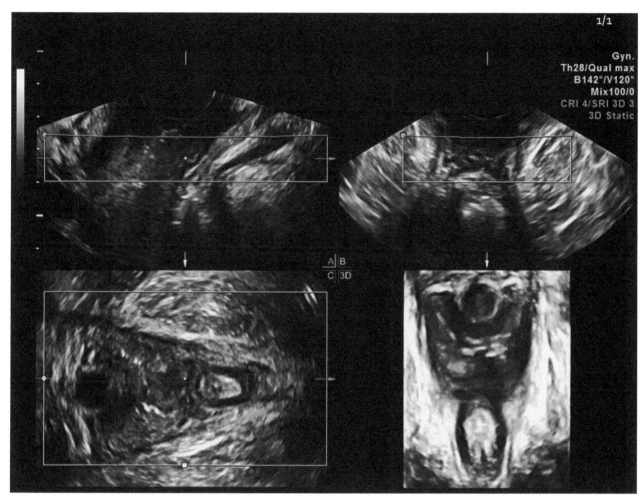

Fig. 309

CASE 144, FIGURE 310

27. Fig. 310 demonstrates a transabdominal image using a 2–5 MHz transducer of the left ovary on a peri-menopausal 50-year-old patient with a clinically palpated left lower quadrant adnexal mass that is larger than 8 × 10 cm using a 2–5 MHz transabdominal exam. What is the depth of view for this image?
   a. 11 cm
   b. 12 cm

28. Fig. 310. Though there are two normal-appearing follicles seen on this cut (red arrows), the overall echo pattern of the ovary is best described as which of the following:
   a. Heterogeneous; complex primarily cystic in appearance with posterior acoustic enhancement and irregular contour
   b. Heterogeneous; complex primarily solid in appearance with posterior acoustic enhancement and irregular contour
   c. Heterogeneous; complex primarily cystic in appearance with posterior acoustic shadowing and smooth contour
   d. Heterogeneous; complex primarily solid in appearance with posterior acoustic shadowing and smooth contour

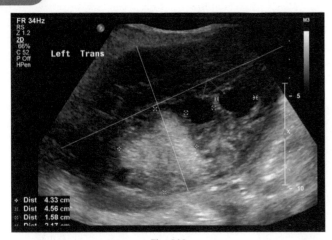

Fig. 310

CASE 145, FIGURE 311

29. As a sonohysterogram is nearly completed, there will nearly always be residual infused saline within the cervical canal during which the examiner can rule out the presence of additional findings as the EV transducer is removed. Fig. 311 demonstrates a ML sagittal lower uterine segment/cervical image using a 4–8 MHz EV transducer on a 42-year-old patient found to have endometrial polyps during the procedure. The presence of an irregular elongated hyperechoic cervical lesion (red arrow) is found on a patient, which is well visualized by the residual fluid and thought to represent a cervical polyp.

    An additional incidental finding is noted on the same image (white arrow). What question should be asked of the patient's history? _____

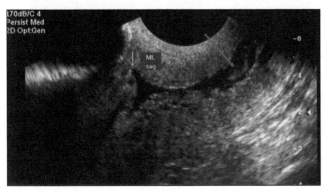

Fig. 311

CASE 146, FIGURES 312–314

30. Figs. 312–314 are transperineal images, using a 6–12 MHz EV transducer, of a 54-year-old patient with urgency and stress urinary incontinence. She thinks she had a suburethral sling in 2003, but she is unsure. With her uncertainty regarding whether she had a sling placed 17 years ago, the goal of the exam is to confirm its presence as well as assess the anatomy to explain the reason for her symptoms. Fig. 312 is a 3D volume set of the pelvic floor. Answer the following questions with Yes or No.

    a. The urethra appears within normal limits in contour. _____

    b. The bladder is full. _____

    c. The center reference point is placed at the distal urethra. _____

    d. The C plane (screen bottom left and right) is an axial urethral cut. _____

    e. There is no evidence on this image of a suburethral sling. _____

31. Fig. 313 demonstrates a second 3D volume set taken at a plane slightly off midline of the pelvic floor on the same patient at which a hyperechoic focus is now seen posterior to the distal urethra on the A plane (gold arrow). Which of the other two orthogonal planes is an image of the bulk of focus (consistent with mesh) seen—B or C plane? _____

32. Notice on Fig. 314 that the transperineal transducer is steeply angled back to the mesh so that the 3D volume sweep's green line of reference can be moved right down to the mesh to create a better approach for the rendered image, which now displays the entire mesh from side to side (red arrows), whereas the B plane only demonstrates the left arm. At what level is the sling relative to the urethra—proximal, mid, or distal? _____

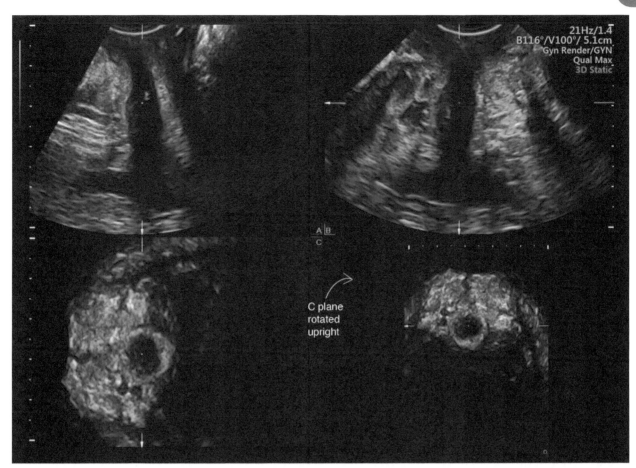

Fig. 312

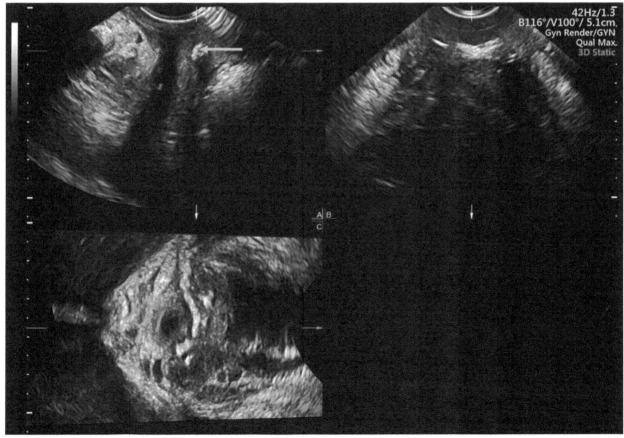

Fig. 313

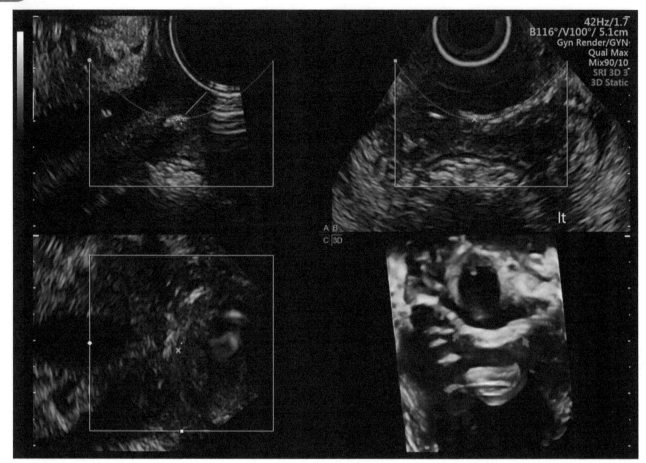

Fig. 314

CASE 147, FIGURE 315

33. Fig. 315 demonstrates instrumentation information available on the ultrasound screen, which can be seen during and post exam on every saved image. This is quite varied in location among the ultrasound systems, but taking the time to see where these are on your system will give you tools to check and enhance the exam. Check out the screen and answer the following questions.
   a. FR is how many times per second the image changes. What is the FR? _____
   b. Is the vascularity seen using Color Power Doppler of Doppler Color Flow? _____
   c. What is the frequency of the transducer? _____
   d. What are two ways to see the depth of view on this screen? _____

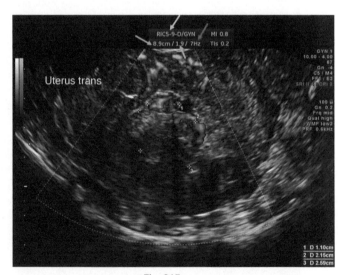

Fig. 315

CASE 148, FIGURE 316

34. Parts A and B of Fig. 316 are two anal sphincter complex (ASC) images using a 5–9 MHz EV transducer. Answer the following questions.
    a. Are these images transperineal or endoanal? _____

    b. Is the internal anal sphincter intact at these levels? _____

c. Is there elevation of the central mucosa at these levels? _____
d. Do the 12, 3, 6, and 9 OC locations appear symmetric on image A? _____
e. Do the 12, 3, 6, and 9 OC locations appear symmetric on image B? _____
f. Which is at the distal ASC complex—A or B? _____

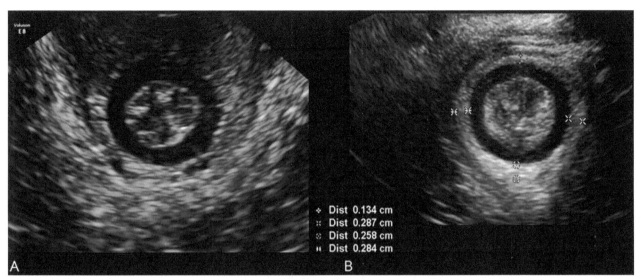

Fig. 316

CASE 149, FIGURE 317

35. Fig. 317 represents 3D rendered images of the bladder luminal wall of two asymptomatic patients using a 6–12 MHz EV transducer. Sometimes idiopathic mild trabeculations can be identified on an asymptomatic patient when a transperineal pelvic floor examination is being performed. Which of the images demonstrates mild trabeculations—A, B, or both? _____

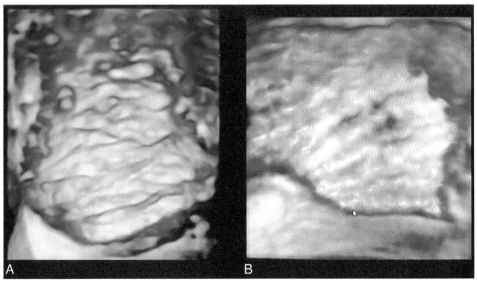

Fig. 317

CASE 150, FIGURE 318

36. Fig. 318 is a 3D volume set of a 63-year-old patient using a 5–9 MHz EV transducer. At which of the orthogonal planes (A, B, or C) is the urethral length measured? _____

37. Is the center reference point at the proximal, mid, or distal urethra? _____

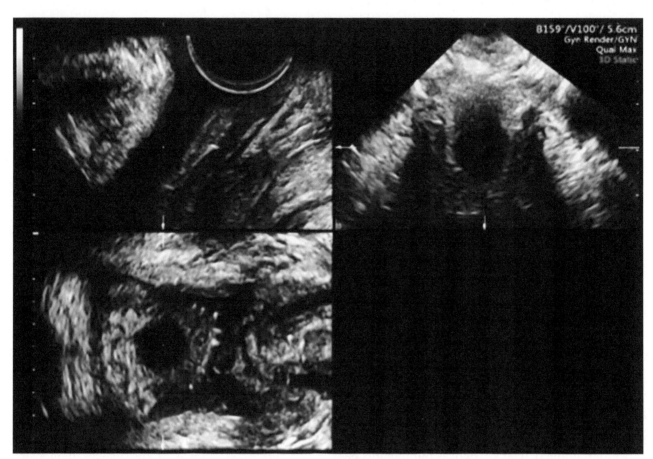

Fig. 318

Case Reviews 151–165

TOPIC 9, FIGURE 319

1. Fig. 319. Topic: Information on the 3D Volume Set Screen Is Abundant.

A good 3D volume set will provide much information all on one screen. This is a transperineal 3D volume set with a rendered view of a 75-year-old patient who has trouble voiding and a history of a urethral sling placement for urinary incontinence. A second rendered image is shown (screen right).

The acquisition A plane is a midsagittal cut of the urethra, which is compressed anteriorly at the mid-distal segment by the echogenic sling (yellow arrow), causing a widened proximal urethra (red arrow), a very thin mid segment, and a short distal segment (white arrow). The B plane is posterior to the urethra and demonstrates a coronal cut of the sling at the center reference point (CRP) of the A plane. The C plane is an axial cut of the sling, seen posterior to the compressed urethra (green arrow). Remember to take advantage of the vertical and horizontal partial lines along the edges of the images, which would intersect at the CRP.

The green square icon seen along the side of the A and B images indicates the right side of the patient. The green diamond on image C indicates the anterior direction. The green line of reference is brought down *to* the CRP to provide the best rendered view of the mid-distal sling placement.

The screen bottom right image of the volume set is the rendered view of the urethra and the sling posterior to it. Notice the atypical appearance of the compressed urethra (green arrow) on the 3D rendered images. This compression results in the widened proximal urethra and the markedly enlarged bladder, partially seen as prolapsing inferior-posteriorly.

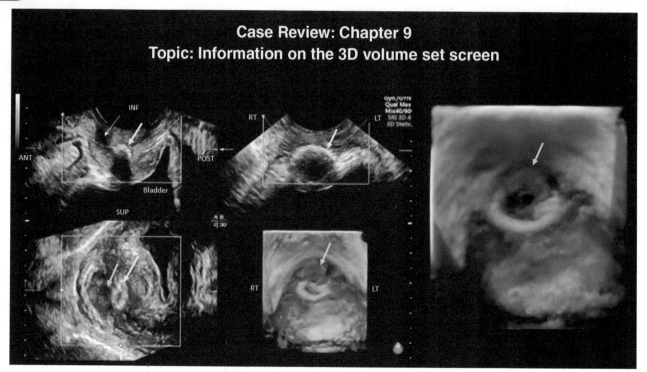

Case Review: Chapter 9
Topic: Information on the 3D volume set screen

Fig. 319

CASE 151, FIGURES 320 AND 321

2. Fig. 320 is a transperineal 3D volume set of a 54-year-old patient with stress urinary incontinence, which had worsened since a mid-urethral sling placed at an outside institution was "resected."

   The orthogonal planes of the 3D volume set as related to the urethra are relative to what the examiner uses as the original acquisition sweep plane. In this case, the volume sweep is made at a midline (ML) sagittal cut; therefore, the A plane image is a sagittal cut through the urethra.

   As shown on Fig. 320, the B plane is perpendicular to the A plane (light blue vertical line) at the CRP. It is coronal on the patient and posterior to the urethra. The C plane is coronal to the A plane, as seen at the red horizontal line. It is axial on the patient at the proximal urethra.

   From Figs. 320 and 321, assess the overall appearance of the urethra on the orthogonal planes as well as the 3D rendered urethral image.
   a. Is the urethra irregular or smooth in contour?

   _____

   b. Is there evidence of full, partial, or no residual hyperechoic mesh? _____
   c. Remember, the top of the screen on a transperineal image is inferior, so the bottom of the screen is superior on the patient. The 3D *rendered* image (bottom right) is as if the viewer is looking from above into the green line of reference on A and B planes, which is "up" the urethra and superior on the patient (toward the proximal urethral

level). Screen left of the rendered image (bottom right) is the patient's right side. Is the residual mesh seen on the rendered image primarily to the left, at the central, or to the right of ML location(s)? _____

3. On Fig. 320, note that the CRP is seen on all three planes at the residual mesh location (white arrow). Where the CRP is placed is the examiner's decision, depending on the purpose of the specific volume planes. On the A plane, is the CRP seen posterior to the proximal, mid, or distal aspect of the urethra?

   _____

4. Moving the CRP is the examiner's role at the time of the exam depending on the desired visualization of a specific area of interest. It can also be moved at the 3D workstation post exam to move through the saved volume. Why is the mesh seen but the urethra *not seen* on the B plane?
   a. It is not seen because the B cut is anterior to the urethra as seen on the A plane by the CRP location.
   b. It is not seen because the B cut is to the right of the urethra as seen on the A plane by the CRP location.
   c. It is not seen because the B cut is posterior to the urethra as seen on the A plane by the CRP location.
   d. It is not seen because the B cut is to the left of the urethra as seen on the A plane by the CRP location.

5. Does the mesh appear symmetric or asymmetric on the 3D rendered image? _____

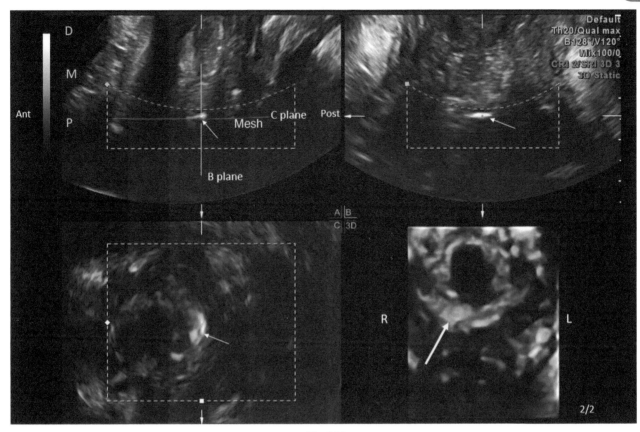

Fig. 320

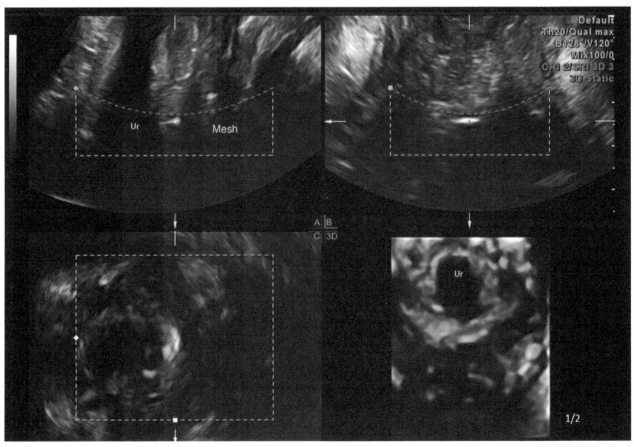

Fig. 321

CASE 152, FIGURES 322–327

6. Figs. 322–327 are endovaginal (EV) images, using a 3–9 MHz transducer, of a 26-year-old who was diagnosed with a right-sided 4 × 4 cm tubo-ovarian abscess (TOA) from an ultrasound exam done at an outside institution 6 weeks ago. Her last menstrual period (LMP) was 8 days ago. Fig. 322 is a midsagittal uterine image. There is minimal posterior cul de sac (PCDS) free fluid (FF) present on today's exam (blue arrow) compared with the last exam, at which time there was moderate FF noted. The left ovary appears within normal limits (WNL) (Fig. 323). Answer the following questions. In what position is the uterus—anteverted (AV), retroverted (RV), anteflexed (AF), retroflexed (RF), or neutral?
   a. AV
   b. RV
   c. AV, AF
   d. Neutral
   e. RV, RF

7. In what phase of the cycle is the endometrium?
   a. Early proliferative
   b. Late proliferative
   c. Mid-cycle
   d. Early secretory
   e. Late secretory

8. Figs. 324 and 325. Which of the following best describes the measured 3.51 × 2.28 × 2.45 cm component of the right ovary that measures smaller than the previously reported size of 4 × 4 cm?
   a. Oval-shaped, thick-walled intraovarian lesion with hyperechoic central area
   b. Thick-walled intraovarian lesion with heterogeneous hypoechoic central area
   c. Round, thick-walled intraovarian lesion with anechoic central area
   d. Oval-shaped, thin-walled intraovarian homogeneous hypoechoic central lesion

9. Figs. 326 and 327. No Doppler spectral waveform, including the resistive index (RI) of the area of concern, was obtained on the first exam. Which Color Power Doppler description below best characterizes the intraovarian lesion?
   a. Diffusely vascular with high RI
   b. Centrally vascular with low RI
   c. Peripherally vascular with a low RI
   d. Peripherally vascular with a high RI

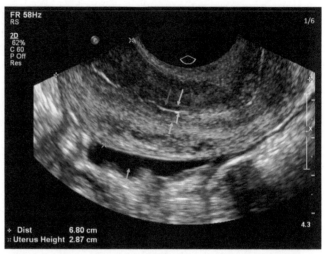

Fig. 322

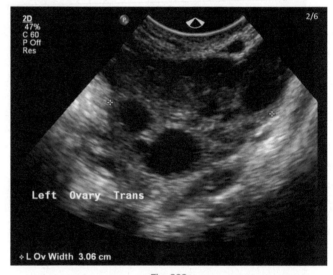

Fig. 323

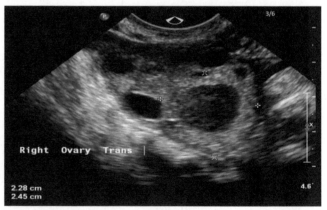

Fig. 324

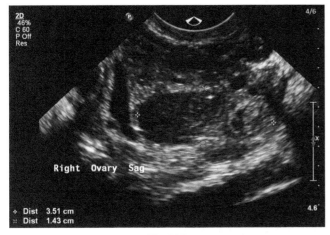

Fig. 325

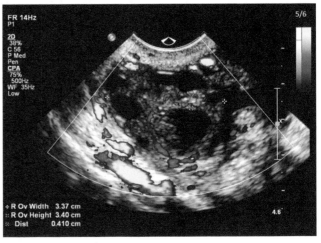

Fig. 326

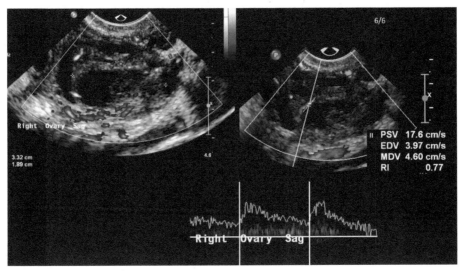

Fig. 327

CASE 153, FIGURES 328–331

10. Figs. 328–331 demonstrate EV 2D and 3D volume set images, using a 5–9 MHz EV transducer, of the retroverted uterus on a 45-year-old female with a history of pelvic pain. The patient has a negative human chorionic gonadotropin (hCG). Her LMP was 19 days ago. In what position is the uterus? _____

11. In what phase of the endometrial cycle is the sonographic appearance?
    a. Post-menses
    b. Proliferative
    c. Mid-cycle
    d. Secretory

12. Fig. 328 demonstrates an oval anechoic structure labeled "A". Fig. 329 is the 3D volume set with the acquisition sweep at midline sagittal and the CRP placed at the central endometrium. Now an additional anechoic structure labeled "B" measuring less than 1 mm in diameter is seen. Are the anechoic structures identified as "A" and "B" intraendometrial or at the endometrial/myometrial interface? _____

13. Fig. 329. The 3D rendered image has been removed. The "C" plane of the 3D volume set has been rotated counterclockwise (curved arrow) to be upright on the Z-axis. What additional finding (green arrows) is noted?
    a. Peri-ovarian free fluid
    b. Bilateral diffuse ovarian follicles
    c. Tortuous peripheral vasculature
    d. Normal uterine appearance

14. How does the Color Power Doppler, as seen on Fig. 330, support the negative hCG? _____

15. By moving the CRP on the C plane to structure A on Fig. 331, all three planes visualize the larger lesion. Which of the following is the best sonographic diagnosis for these findings? _____
    a. Endometrial cavity free fluid
    b. Resorbing gestational sac
    c. Endometrial cysts
    d. Spiral artery
    e. Adenomyosis
    f. Intrauterine pregnancy (IUP)

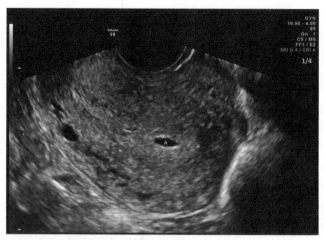

Fig. 328

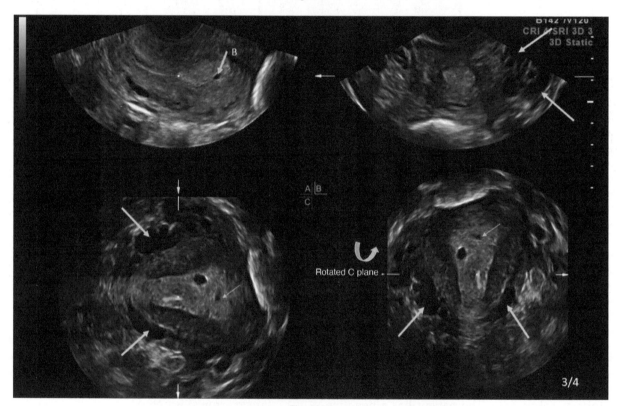

Fig. 329

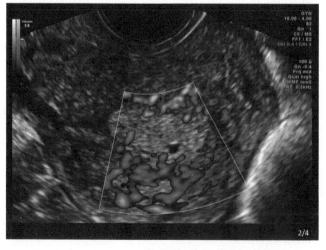

Fig. 330

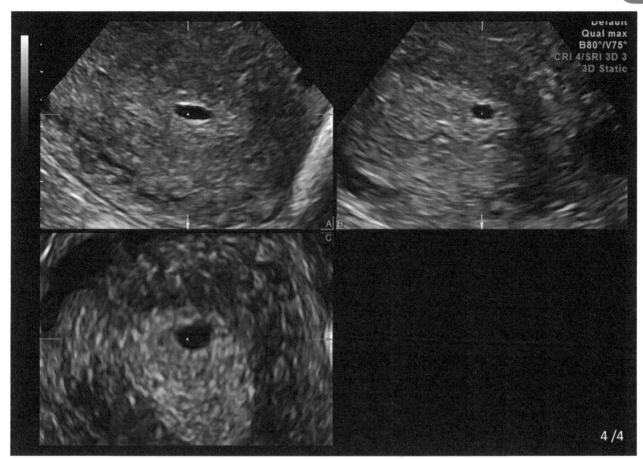

Fig. 331

CASE 154, FIGURES 332 AND 333

16. Figs. 332 and 333 represent a 3D volume set using a 5–9 MHz EV transducer on a Gyn patient to assess intrauterine device (IUD) placement. The B and C planes perfectly demonstrate the arms of the IUD at the fundal end of the endometrial cavity. Notice that the CRP (green arrows) is visualized at the IUD on Fig. 332 located between the two arms (B and C planes). In what position is the uterus—anteverted (AV), retroverted (RV), anteflexed (AF), retroflexed (RF), or neutral?
    a. AV, RF
    b. Neutral
    c. RV
    d. RV, RF

17. Fig. 332. Why is the IUD stem not seen on this volume set? _____

18. Identify the labeled structures.
    1 _____
    2 _____
    3 _____

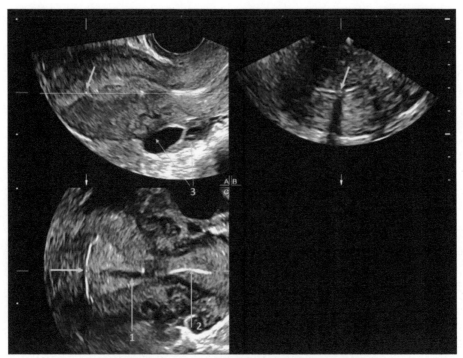

Fig. 332

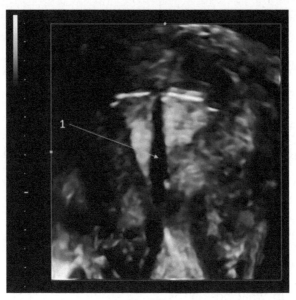

Fig. 333

CASE 155, FIGURES 334–337

19. On a rare occasion, an unusual exam will present itself when 3D assessment will be the only vehicle to detail the findings. Figs. 334–337 are those of a 60-year-old postmenopausal patient visiting from China who was referred for an enlarged uterus and suspected central pelvic mass. The ovaries were visualized and appeared WNL and are not shown. Fig. 334 is a midsagittal image of an enlarged heterogeneous uterus using a 6–12 MHz EV transducer. The length and anteroposterior diameter are measured on the 2D sagittal image. Measure the transverse width on the coronal C plane of Fig. 335 between the two gold lines and calculate the uterine volume using the Fig. 334 and 335 measurements. _____ cm³.

20. The endometrium was not definitively visualized throughout the exam because of the presence of diffuse myomatous lesions of various sizes and echo patterns, especially at the mid to posterior uterine aspect. Findings are consistent with leiomyomata.

Noted from the beginning of the 2D exam was a hyperechoic curvilinear structure seen at the lower uterine segment (LUS; white arrows), as seen on Figs. 335–337. Subsequent 3D volume repositioning of the center reference point onto the hyperechoic structure on the volume images (Figs. 336 and 337), and movement of the green line of reference (LOR) through the volume set on A and B planes to the hyperechoic focus brings it into view on all three planes. Additionally, moving the LOR from lateral to medial on Fig. 337 allows a rendered appearance of the entire round structure. What does #1 represent on Fig. 337 at the A plane, C plane, and rendered images? _____

a. Nonspecific ovary
b. Nabothian cysts
c. Left ovary
d. Cervix
e. Posterior LUS
f. Right ovary

21. Fig. 337 demonstrates green diamond- and square-shaped icons at the orthogonal plane edges to help determine direction, especially in unusual cases like this. The diamond and square icons are the same direction in the volume set, no matter what planes are presented.

    The transducer is in the vagina, so the diamond on all planes is inferior.

    The C plane is a coronal cut through the LUS, so the square is anterior on the patient. Which of the following is the best description of the rendered structure image?

a. 4-cm hyperechoic round structure within the displaced lower left endometrium
b. 2-cm hyperechoic round structure within the displaced lower left endometrium
c. 4-cm hyperechoic round structure within the displaced lower right endometrium
d. 2-cm hyperechoic round structure within the displaced lower right endometrium

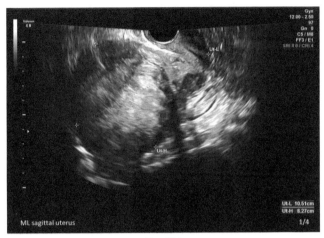

Fig. 334

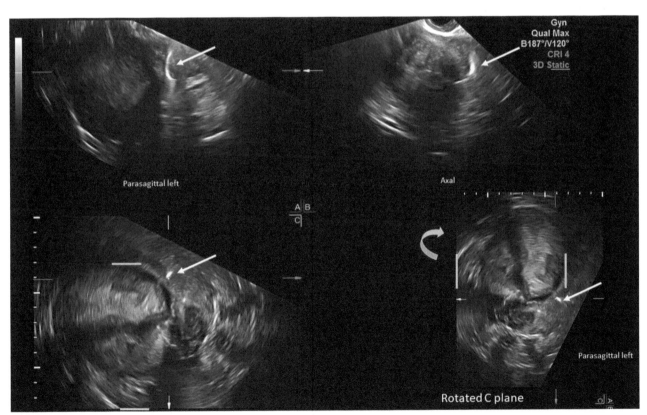

Fig. 335

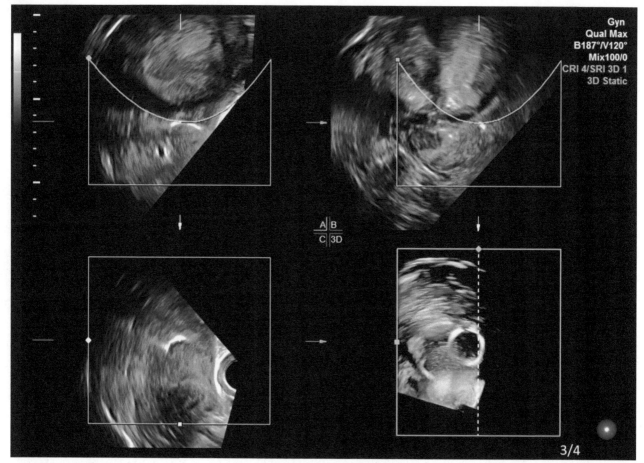

Fig. 336

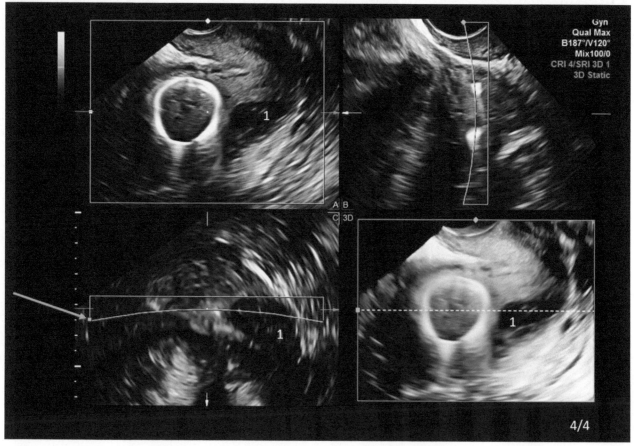

Fig. 337

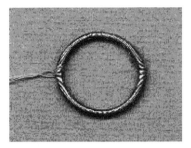

Fig. 337, cont'd

CASE 156, FIGURE 338

22. Fig. 338 is a midline sagittal image of the uterus on a patient with a history of menorrhagia following a sonohysterogram. Based on the gold arrowed finding, which was not seen on the pre-procedure midsagittal image, which of the following is true?
    a. The right tube is blocked.
    b. The left tube is blocked.
    c. At least one tube is patent.
    d. Both tubes are patent.

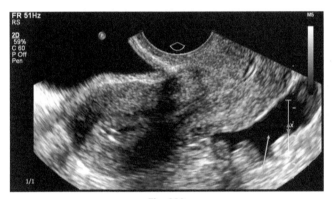

Fig. 338

CASE 157, FIGURES 339–341

23. Figs. 339–341 are images from a 3D volume set of a 34-year-old patient with menorrhagia, or abnormal uterine bleeding. Her LMP was 2 weeks ago.

    At the top of this and any vendor's image, there will be some location where the transducer frequency, depth of view, level of read zoom magnification, and frame rate (FR) are provided, as seen on Fig. 339 (white arrow).

    The top line indicates what transducer is being used, which is the 5–9 MHz EV curvilinear transducer. The *bottom left* is the depth of view (how deep the field of view is from the transducer to the bottom of the image) at 6.7 cm, even though the image is zoomed and the calipers along the side are not all seen; the *center* depicts the amount of magnification of the original image at 1.4x; and the *right* is the FR or the number of times the

image is changed per second (Hz). If you learn where these tools are on the screen, it will help in your assessment confidence.

The appearance of the endometrium appears heterogeneous and indicates the presence of multiple intracavitary lesions. One can, however, suggest in which phase of her cycle she is by the varied appearances of the basal and functional components of the endometrium.
    a. Early proliferative
    b. Late proliferative
    c. Mid-cycle
    d. Early secretory
    e. Late secretory

24. By moving the center reference point to the central endometrial cavity on Fig. 339, the appearance of lesion complexity is enhanced on all three planes. To what are the green arrows pointing on the rendered image of Fig. 340?
    a. Basal layer of the endometrium
    b. Functional layer of the endometrium
    c. Free fluid within the endometrial cavity
    d. Myometrial/endometrial interface

25. Is the echogenicity of the intracavity lesion complex hypoechoic, isoechoic, or hyperechoic compared with the endometrium? ____

26. Is the intracavitary lesion smooth and singular or irregular and multilobulated in contour? ____

27. Fig. 341 is one cut of the Color Power Doppler of the endometrium with the gray scale post-processed to enhance the lesions. Which of the following is true?
    a. The endometrium demonstrates several feeder vessels into hypoechoic lesions.
    b. The endometrium demonstrates a normal smooth homogeneous echo pattern with no increased intralesion vascularity.
    c. The endometrium demonstrates a heterogeneous pattern with several lesions and some intralesion vascularity.
    d. The endometrium contains several small submucosal leiomyomata with peripheral hypervascularity.

28. What is the most likely diagnosis for these findings? ____

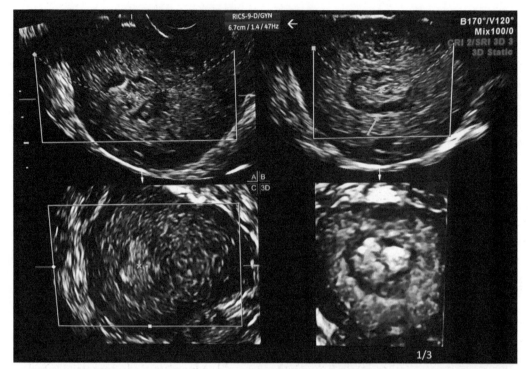

Fig. 339

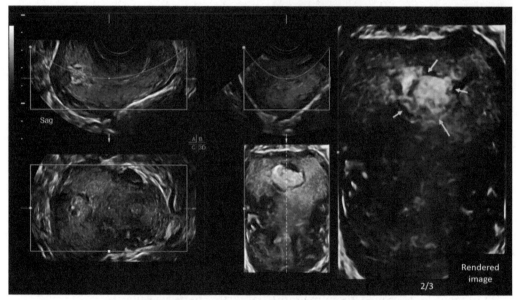

Fig. 340

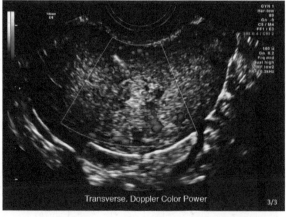

Fig. 341

CASE 158, FIGURE 342

29. Fig. 342 demonstrates an adnexal mass on a patient with left lower quadrant pain using a 4–8 MHz EV transducer. The right ovary appears normal and is not demonstrated here. Which of the following is the best description of the left ovary?
    a. The enlarged left ovary demonstrates a central homogeneous low-level echo pattern.
    b. The enlarged left ovary demonstrates a complex primarily cystic appearance.
    c. The enlarged left ovary demonstrates a central complex primarily solid appearance.
    d. The enlarged left ovary demonstrates a heterogeneous echo pattern with an irregular hyperechoic mass.

30. Fig. 342. Which segmental aspect is more worrisome of the mass—A or B?

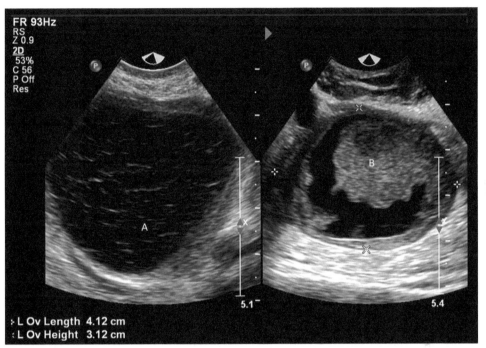

Fig. 342

CASE 159, FIGURES 343 AND 344

31. Figs. 343 and 344 are the C plane (coronal, in this case) of the uterus on an exam to assess the intrauterine contraceptive device in the absence of lost strings. The C plane in the volume set is a coronal cut through the A plane (which is midsagittal) that looks horizontal; so, with rotation on the Z-axis, the coronal plane is now upright. Is the IUD located within the central endometrial cavity? _____

32. Can you see evidence of the strings on Fig. 343, Fig. 344, neither, or both? _____

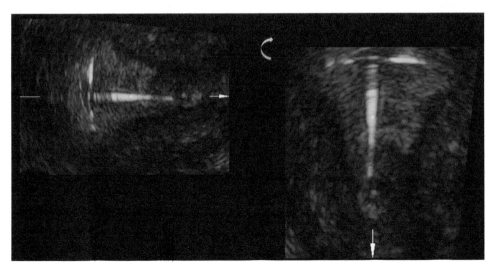

Fig. 343

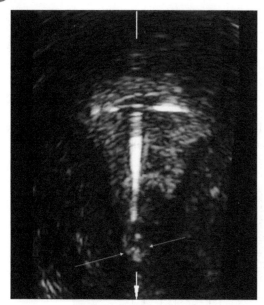

Fig. 344

CASE 160, FIGURES 345 AND 346

33. Figs. 345 and 346 are images, using a 5–9 MHz EV transducer, of a 30-year-old with a long-term history of menometrorrhagia, or abnormal uterine bleeding (AUB). The 3D volume set of the uterus and endometrium demonstrates a secretory endometrium with a scant amount of free fluid within the endometrial cavity (gold arrows). The endometrium appears relatively homogeneous at first; however, 2D Color Power Doppler images (Fig. 346) and high-contrast post-processing demonstrate the vascular flow and echo patterns of the endometrium to confirm which of the following?

   a. No color flow is depicted within the heterogeneous endometrium.
   b. Abnormal flow is depicted centrally into the heterogeneous endometrium.
   c. Abnormal peripheral flow of the homogeneous endometrium is noted.
   d. Normal diffuse flow within the homogeneous endometrium is noted.

34. Which of the following is the most likely etiology for this appearance?
   a. Endometrial carcinoma
   b. Degenerated submucosal leiomyoma
   c. Endometrial polyps
   d. Mid-cycle endometrial cavity free fluid

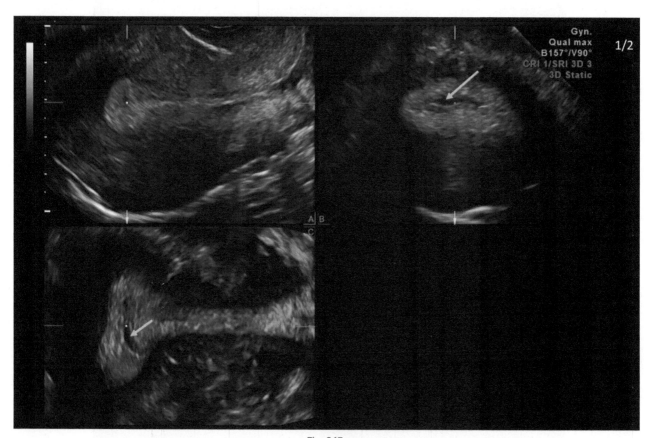

Fig. 345

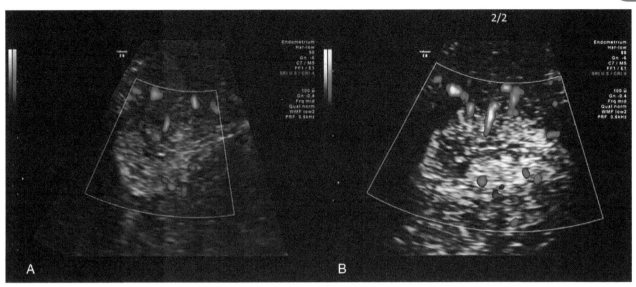

Fig. 346

CASE 161, FIGURE 347

35. Fig. 347 is a magnified image of the internal anal sphincter (IAS).
    a. What is the frame rate of this exam? _____
    b. Based on the frame rate and the image size, is this more likely to be a read zoomed image or a write zoomed image? _____
    c. The IAS is disrupted from where to where (as if on a clock)? _____
    d. Is there elevation of the central mucosa? _____
    e. To what do the gold arrows point? _____
    f. At what level is this cut—proximal, mid, or distal? _____

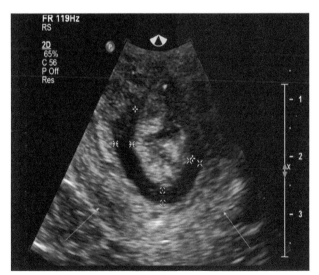

Fig. 347

CASE 162, FIGURES 348–352

36. Figs. 348–352 represent findings, using a 5–9 MHz EV transducer, of a 40-year-old patient with a history of menorrhagia, or AUB, who was clinically found to have an enlarged uterus. Both ovaries appear normal and are not presented. In what phase of the menstrual cycle is the endometrium?
    a. Post-menses
    b. Proliferative
    c. Mid-cycle
    d. Secretory

37. A large oblong-shaped myomatous lesion is easily identified at the mid-posterior segment of the uterus, finding consistent with leiomyoma. Is the myoma large enough to affect the contour of the endometrium? _____

38. Figs. 349 and 350 reveal a post-processed and chroma image of the endometrial thickness measurement where a small round hyperechoic endometrial lesion is seen, which was not as appreciated on the initial gray-scale midsagittal cut. As related to the basal layer of the endometrium, the lesion appears:
    a. Hypoechoic
    b. Isoechoic
    c. Hyperechoic

39. A 3D volume set of the lesion with the center reference point (green arrows) brought to the lesion is seen on Fig. 351 before the rendered image is obtained. Figs. 351 and 352 demonstrate the well-circumscribed lesion on the rendered image. When the green line of reference is brought to the endometrial interface on the A and B planes, the quality of the rendered image (Fig. 352) becomes successfully heightened. The most likely sonographic diagnosis is:
    a. Endometrial polyp
    b. Subserosal leiomyoma
    c. Endometrial carcinoma
    d. Submucosal leiomyoma

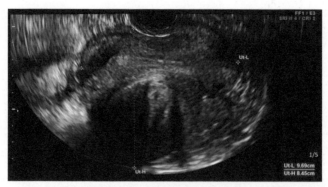

Fig. 348

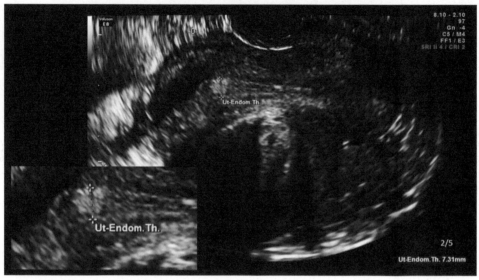

Fig. 349

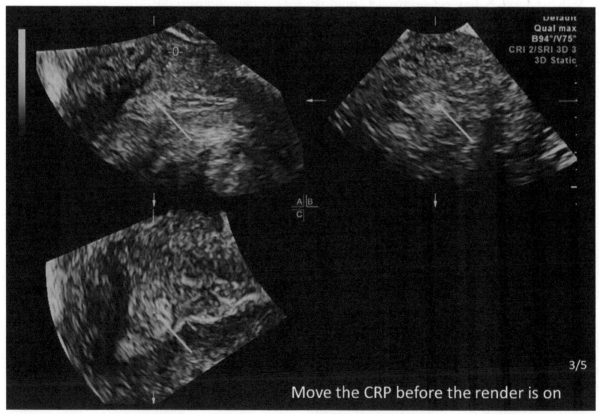

Fig. 350

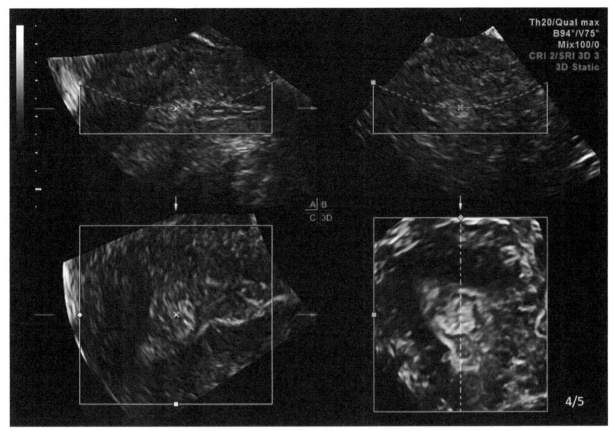

Fig. 351

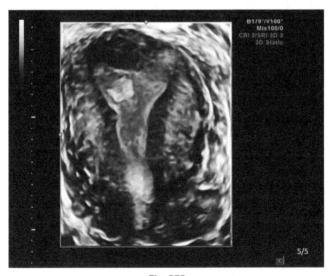

Fig. 352

CASE 163, FIGURES 353–356

40. A 45-year-old patient was referred for a second opinion of a 6 × 6 cm adnexal mass that was diagnosed as a "simple cyst" at another imaging center. Fig. 353 is a 3D volume set using a 5–9 MHz EV transducer of the mass with the CRP seen in the expected original middle-of-the-volume sweep location. With a parallel shift through the entire volume to the back wall of the mass, Fig. 354 demonstrates the presence of luminal wall irregularities and several punctate echogenic foci (green arrows) not appreciated on the initial A, B, and C planes.

An additional 3D volume (Figs. 355 and 356) confirms the irregularities when the CRP was moved to the area of interest along the back wall of the mass (yellow arrow). The acquisition plane (A) is a sagittal cut of the mass; therefore, the B plane is transverse *at* the CRP (on the A plane) and the C plane is coronal to the CRP (on the A plane). X-, Y-, and Z-axis rotations further fine-tuned the render image to create a cleaner surface.

Review the green icons seen on the 3D volume orthogonal planes (Fig. 355) as well as the rendered image (Fig. 356). What direction on the patient is the *diamond* icon (white arrow)?

a. Superior
b. Inferior
c. Right
d. Left
e. Posterior
f. Anterior

41. What direction on the patient is the *square* icon (red arrow)?

    a. Superior
    b. Inferior
    c. Right
    d. Left
    e. Posterior
    f. Anterior

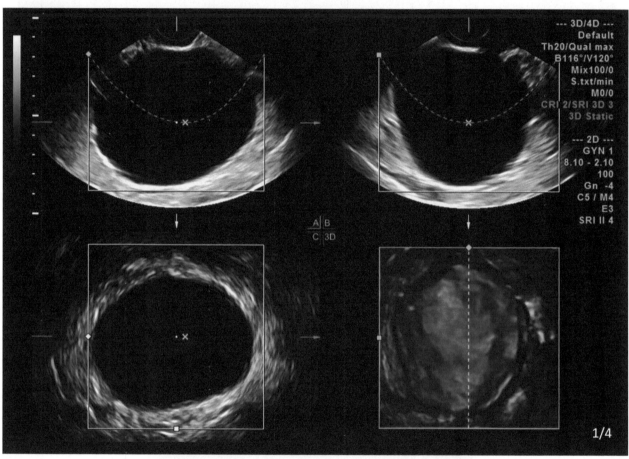

Fig. 353

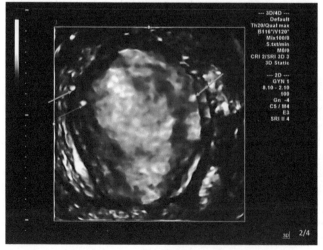

Fig. 354

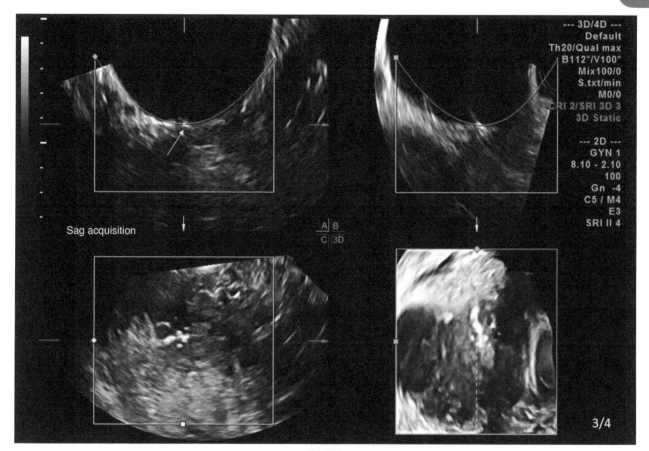

Fig. 355

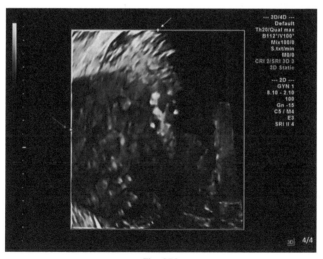

Fig. 356

CASE 164, FIGURE 357

42. Fig. 357 demonstrates three separate 2D axial cuts of mesh found at the anterior vaginal wall on a 51-year-old patient with a history of mesh replacement using a 6–12 MHz EV transducer. Does visualizing the mesh on the axial cuts reveal if the mesh is placed at the mid-urethral level? _____

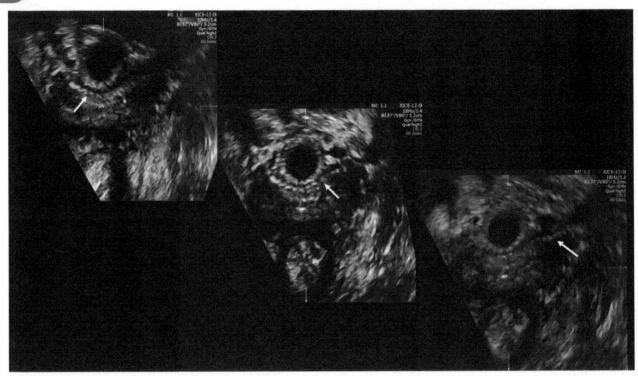

Fig. 357

CASE 165, FIGURE 358

43. Fig. 358 demonstrates two post-void 2D midsagittal images of the urethra using a 6–12 MHz transperineal transducer. The first (screen left) is at rest and the second (screen right) is with cough. With this view, the location of the mesh is clearly seen (gold arrow). At what urethral segment is the mesh located?
   a. Proximal
   b. Proximal-mid
   c. Mid
   d. Mid-distal
   e. Distal

44. With cough, how does the bladder change?
   a. The normal-appearing bladder at rest remains normal in position with cough by immobile mesh.
   b. The normal-appearing bladder at rest distends with cough, bulging posteriorly by immobile mesh.
   c. The normal-appearing bladder at rest remains normal in position with cough by mobile mesh.
   d. The normal-appearing bladder at rest distends with cough, bulging posteriorly by mobile mesh.

45. Based on these findings, is the urethra supported or not supported by the mesh? _____

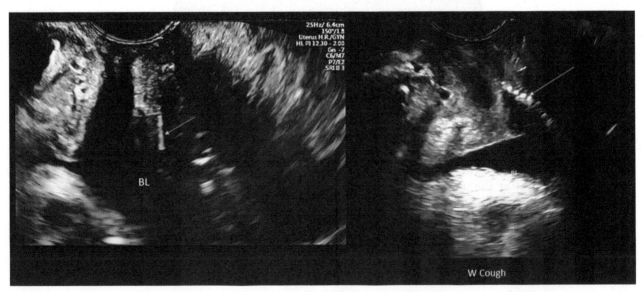

Fig. 358

TOPIC 10, FIGURE 359

1. Fig. 359. Topic: Anal Sphincter Complex (ASC) Color Power Doppler Pulse Repetition Frequency Settings.

Pulse repetition frequency (PRF) indicates the number of ultrasound pulses emitted by the transducer over a designated time frame. It is typically measured as cycles per second or hertz (Hz). The PRF is operator dependent. When using Color Power Doppler, the PRF knob should not be set too low, otherwise image pixels will demonstrate a "blush" to the entire color box, misgauging "flow" where there is none (screen left). Contrarily, if the PRF is set too high, real vascularity will not be present on an image at all, which will underestimate the presence of any vessels and will certainly underrepresent abnormal vascularity (screen right). When the PRF is set appropriately, clear presence of real abnormal flow will be seen (gold arrow).

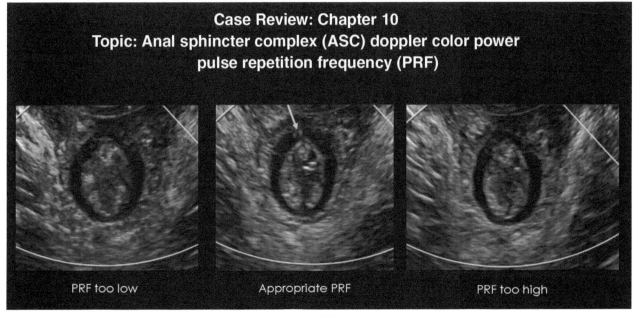

Case Review: Chapter 10
Topic: Anal sphincter complex (ASC) doppler color power pulse repetition frequency (PRF)

PRF too low   Appropriate PRF   PRF too high

Fig. 359

CASE 166, FIGURE 360

2. Though the presence of the correctly placed intrauterine device (IUD) is easy to visualize, there is a wide variability in actual IUD location when comparing exams. Figs. 360–362 are each a different IUD case.

Fig. 360 is a 3D volume set using a 6–12 MHz endovaginal (EV) transducer with a rendered image of a recently placed IUD. Answer the following with a Yes or No.

a. Is the stem located centrally? _____

b. Are the arms contained within the endometrial cavity? _____

c. Is the uterus retroverted? _____

d. Is the center reference point seen on all planes with the green line of reference (LOR) at the appropriate place to optimize the IUD on the rendered image? _____

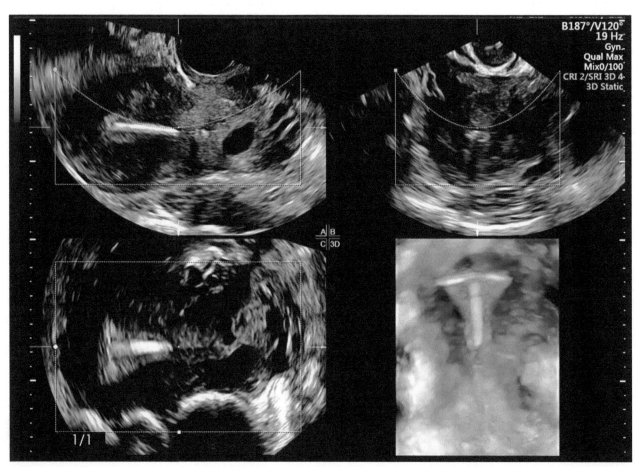

Fig. 360

CASE 167, FIGURE 361

Fig. 361 is a 3D volume set using a 5–9 MHz EV transducer of a postpartum patient who is highly anxious that her recently placed IUD may not be present. Answer the following.

e. Where is the center reference point placed on the volume set to assess the IUD placement? _____

f. Is the IUD placed centrally? _____

g. To what on the C plane are the green arrows pointing? _____

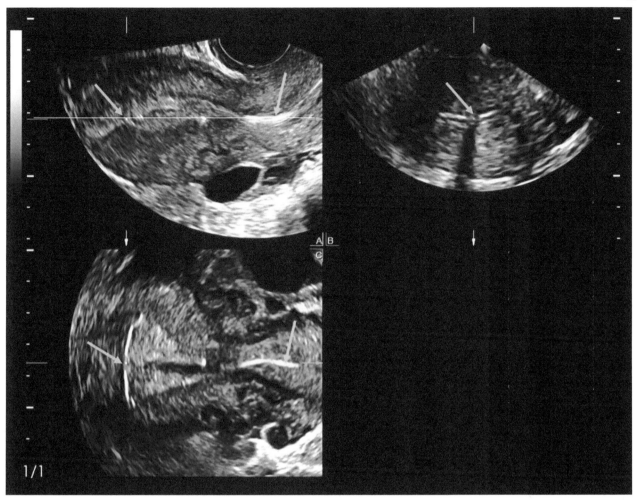

Fig. 361

CASE 168, FIGURE 362

3. Fig. 362 is a 3D volume set on a patient with pelvic discomfort since her IUD was placed. The rendered image has been removed. Which of the following is where the center reference point is placed on the volume set?
   a. It is placed to the right of the midline (ML) central cavity within the right submucosal myometrium.
   b. It is placed to the left of the ML central cavity within the left submucosal myometrium.
   c. It is placed within the central endometrial cavity.
   d. It is placed within the intramural myometrium anterior to the endometrium.

4. Fig. 362. Is the IUD placed centrally within the endometrial cavity?
   a. Yes
   b. No
   c. Cannot tell from these images

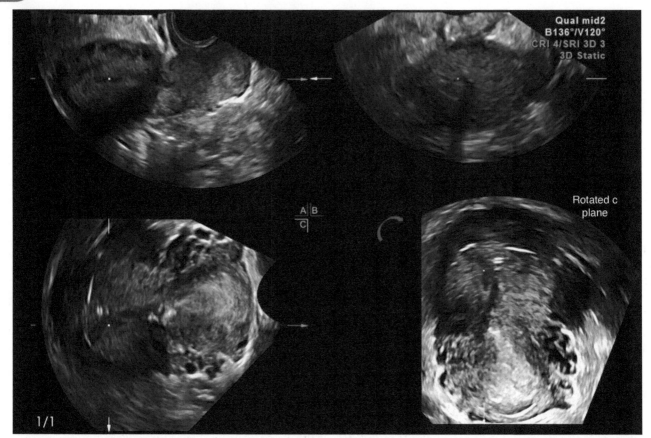

Fig. 362

CASE 169, FIGURES 363–365

5. Figs. 363–365 are images, using a 5–9 MHz EV transducer, of a 33-year-old patient found to have pelvic fullness at her annual exam.
   a. Which ovary has a normal parenchymal echo pattern? _____
   b. Which ovary has abnormally increased size? _____
   c. Which ovary has normal follicular appearance? _____
   d. Which ovary has an irregular contour? _____

6. Color Power Doppler hypervascularity is well visualized on Figs. 364 and 365 of the right ovary. The resistive index at this area (not shown) was 0.71. Is hypervascularity increased at the intraovarian parenchyma or at the hilum? _____
7. Of the following, which is the *least* likely diagnosis for this appearance?
   a. Ovarian carcinoma
   b. Polycystic ovarian syndrome
   c. Dysgerminoma tumor
   d. Sertoli–Leydig cell tumor

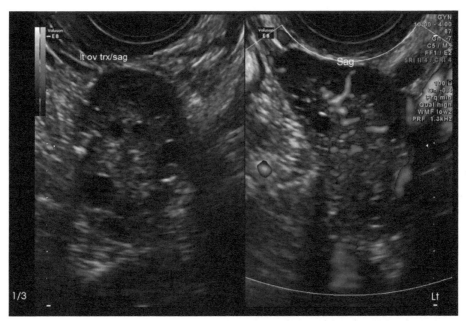

Fig. 363

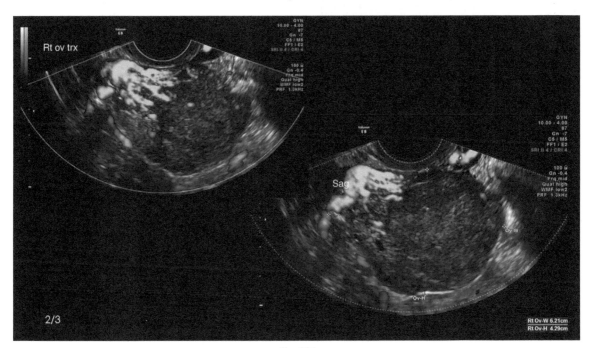

Fig. 364

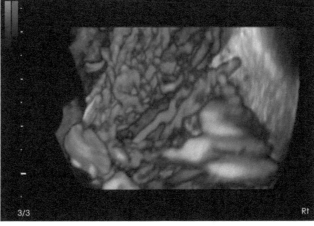

Fig. 365

CASE 170, FIGURE 366

8. Fig. 366 is a mid-uterine transverse image of the lower uterine segment using a 4–8 MHz EV transducer. Which of the following is the most likely etiology for the appearance at the red arrow?
   a. Anterior subserosal leiomyoma
   b. Cesarean section scar
   c. Large endometrial polyp
   d. Septate uterus
   e. Intramural degenerated leiomyoma

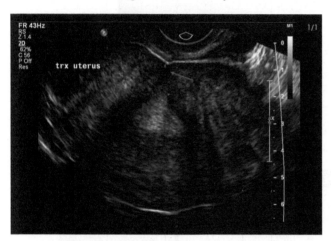

Fig. 366

CASE 171, FIGURES 367–370

9. Figs. 367–370 are transperineal images, using a 6–12 MHz EV transducer, of a 63-year-old patient referred for suspected rectal prolapse that was thought to be compressing the distal vagina anteriorly. Pelvic floor 3D imaging is typically created from a transperineal sweep performed in what plane (the place where the original sweep is placed on the A, B, C volume set).

   Fig. 367. In this case, what plane is the A plane?
   a. Coronal
   b. Sagittal
   c. Transverse

10. Fig. 367. Identify the location of the center reference point (CRP) that is seen on all three orthogonal planes.
    a. Distal urethra
    b. Distal vagina
    c. Mid-urethra
    d. Anal angle of the anal sphincter complex

11. The structures of this volume set to which the arrows are pointing on Figs. 367–370 would be described in terms of:

    Size and shape: Fig. 367. There is an oval-shaped structure that consists of two adjacent components (between gold lines). The hypoechoic trapezoidal-shaped anterior aspect (red arrow) measuring 10 mm and a more hyperechoic oval-shaped posterior aspect (blue arrow) measuring 18 mm together create an oblong heterogeneous structure.

    Echo pattern: All echo comparisons are relative, and in difficult cases like this, the examiner must be careful to appreciate anatomic variations from normal. Since the overall abnormality is heterogeneous (between gold lines), compare the anterior aspect to relative structures and the posterior aspect to relative structures; therefore, the echo pattern is isoechoic where adjacent to the vagina (red arrow) and isoechoic to the bulging central mucosa at the inferior posterior aspect of the bulge (blue arrow). The green arrow points to the connection between the normal central mucosa and the inferior bulge to which it is connected.

    Origin: The origin of the mass structure appears to be rectal with the anterior hypoechoic aspect thought to represent the bulging distal internal anal sphincter (IAS) folded over itself and the posterior hyperechoic aspect representing the bulging central mucosa folded over itself (see between the gold lines on Fig. 367).

    Fig. 368 represents measurements of the anteroposterior diameter of the posterior urethral wall/anterior vagina. Are the measurements symmetric? Yes or No? _____

12. The green LOR on the 3D volume set is brought down to the area of interest on Figs. 368–370. The CRP is also moved from the mid-urethra on Fig. 367 to this IAS/central mucosa interface on Fig. 368, better delineating it on all three orthogonal views. Is there a rectal prolapse? Yes or No? _____

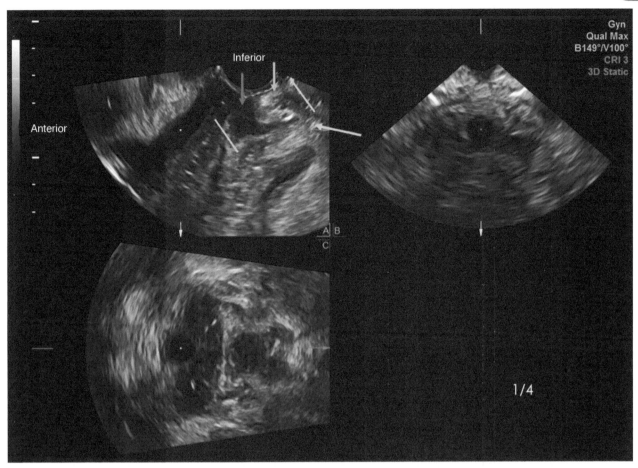

Fig. 367

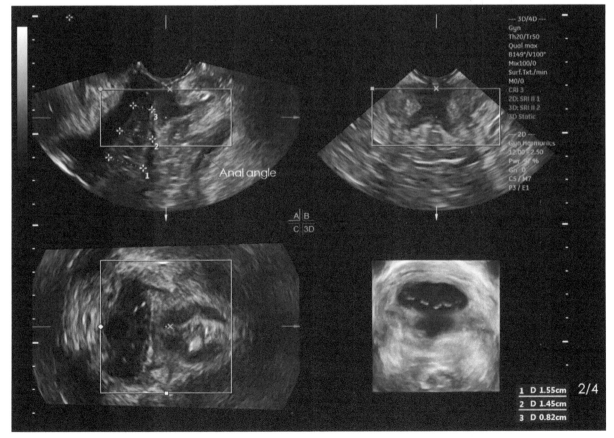

Fig. 368

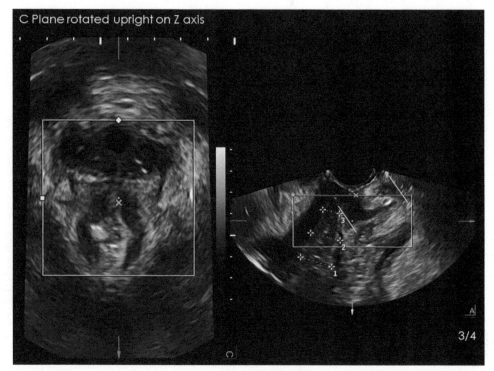

Fig. 369

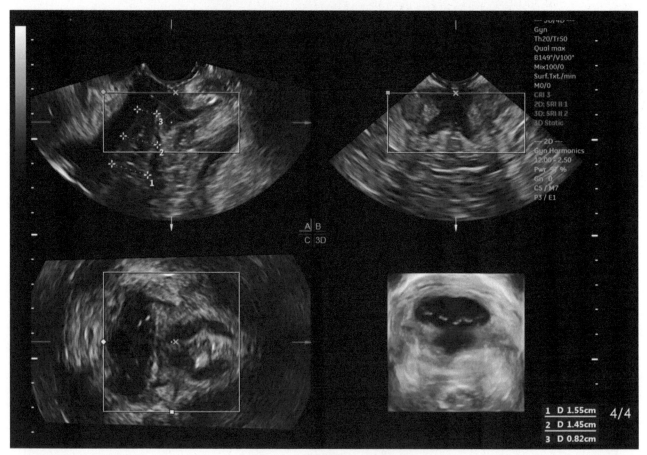

Fig. 370

CASE 172, FIGURES 371–375

13. Figs. 371–375 are those of a 17-year-old with spina bifida who had a recent ultrasound exam and a diagnosed adnexal mass. This follow-up was performed 6 weeks later. The patient is not sexually active. Figs. 371 and 372 demonstrate transabdominal views of normal ovaries, though the bladder was only partially full.

Fig. 373. The 2D imaging suggested a thickened and irregular bladder wall, so a 3D transperineal exam was performed using a 6–12 MHz EV transducer to more optimally assess her bladder (Fig. 374).

When performing a 3D volume sweep of the bladder, make the sweep at least 75 degrees to visualize most of the bladder. By bringing the LOR from the top of the screen down to the area of interest, the rendered image will be enhanced. The red arrows point to the green LOR, which has been brought to the CRP. Fig. 375 is the enlarged 3D rendered image of the bladder wall. Which of the following is the diagnostic finding?

a. Large bladder mass
b. Diffuse bladder wall trabeculations
c. Non-filling of the bladder volume
d. Diffuse bladder wall masses

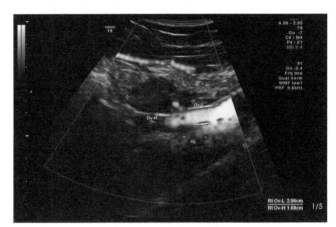

Fig. 371

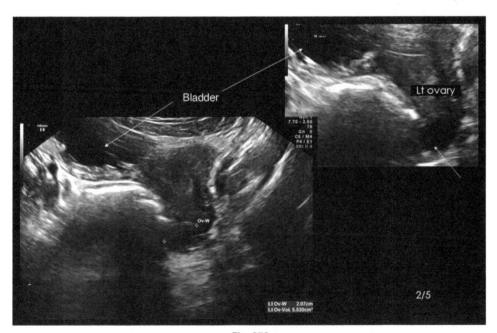

Fig. 372

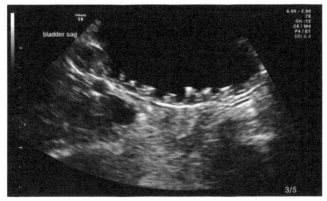

Fig. 373

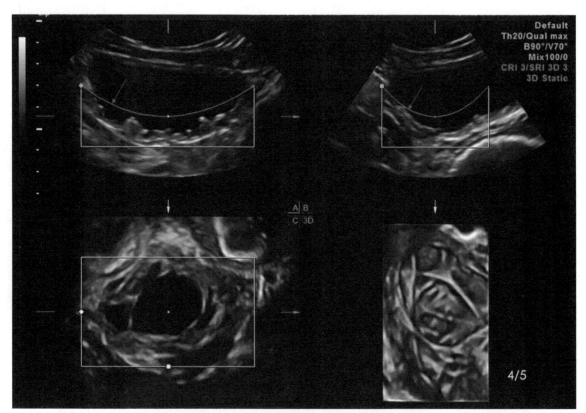

Fig. 374

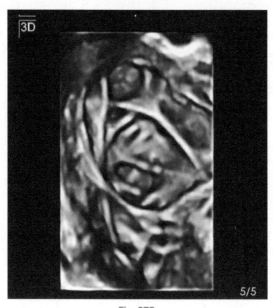

Fig. 375

CASE 173, FIGURES 376–378

14. Figs. 376–378 are those of a 62-year-old woman visiting from Mexico. Though this type of unexpected finding has reduced to nearly zero, the examiner should recognize the appearance of outdated IUDs such as this. Fig. 376 is a 2D mid-sagittal image using a 3–9 MHz EV transducer demonstrating multiple thick echogenic foci within the endometrial cavity with irregular acoustic shadowing seen beyond the endometrium. The patient stated that she had an IUD placed many years ago but had long forgotten it was there. Because of the added volumetric information of a 3D volume sweep, the 3D rendered image, rotated on the Z-axis, better demonstrates which of the following IUD types? (Figs. 377 and 378)

a. ParaGuard
b. Saf-T-coil
c. Dalkon Shield
d. Lippes Loop

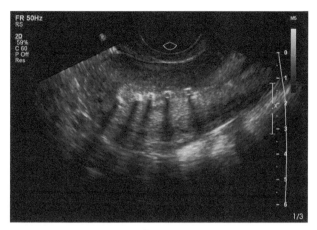

Fig. 376

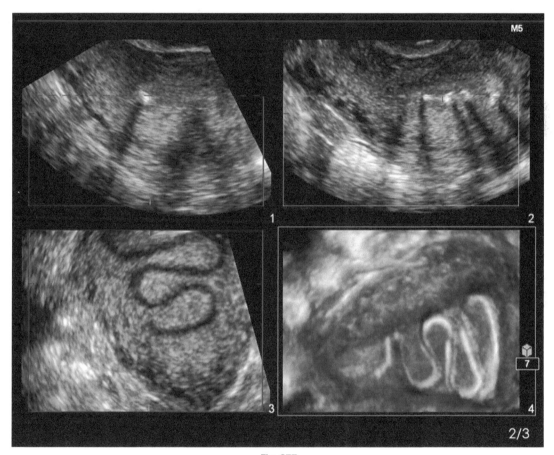

Fig. 377

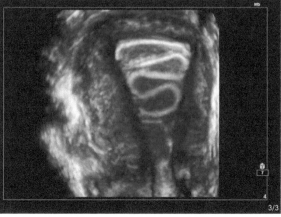

Fig. 378

CASE 174, FIGURE 379

15. Fig. 379 is a post-void 3D volume set of the bladder on a 71-year-old patient with urinary urgency. What is the post-void residual? _____

16. With the center reference point centered at the middle of the bladder and the LOR brought closer to the back of the bladder wall, the 3D volume set well demonstrates overall bladder luminal wall appearance. Which of the following best describes the appearance?
    a. Diffuse mild trabeculations
    b. Smooth bladder luminal wall
    c. Markedly thickened bladder wall
    d. Multiple bladder luminal wall lesions

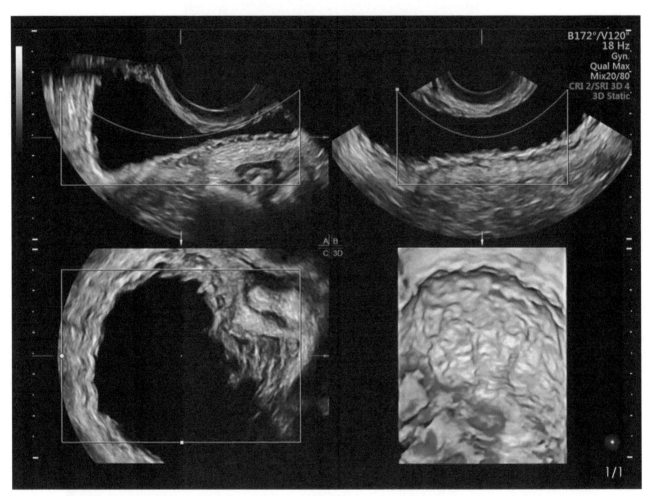

Fig. 379

CASE 175, FIGURE 380

17. Fig. 380 represents midsagittal and mid-uterine transverse images obtained during a sonohysterography procedure using a 4–8MHz EV transducer. The red arrows point to the infused saline. Which of the following is the most likely diagnosis?
    a. Endometrial polyp
    b. Submucosal leiomyoma
    c. Endometrial carcinoma
    d. Intramural leiomyoma

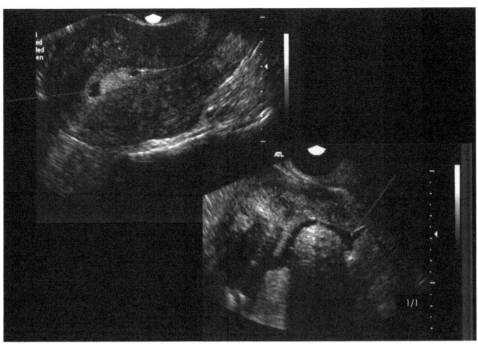

Fig. 380

CASE 176, FIGURE 381

18. Fig. 381 demonstrates a transperineal 3D volume set of the urethra. What each orthogonal plane is for any volume set depends on the examiner's original sweep plane relative to the structure being assessed. Sometimes that plane is the same as the planes of the body, as in this image, but not always. The standard sweep plane of the pelvic floor is thought to be sagittal but may be variable around the world. Additionally, there are times where a different sweep plane initiates new presentation of pathology. Ultimately, volume is volume, so manipulation of multiple sweeps should arrive at the same diagnostic conclusion.

   What is the sweep plane of image A on the urethra? _____

19. Fig. 381. In what cut is the B plane *transecting the urethra* represented by the yellow line? _____

20. What plane is the C plane *transecting the urethra* represented by the red line? _____

21. To what are the blue lines pointing?
    a. Anterior vaginal wall
    b. Air in the vaginal canal
    c. Suburethral sling
    d. Posterior vaginal wall

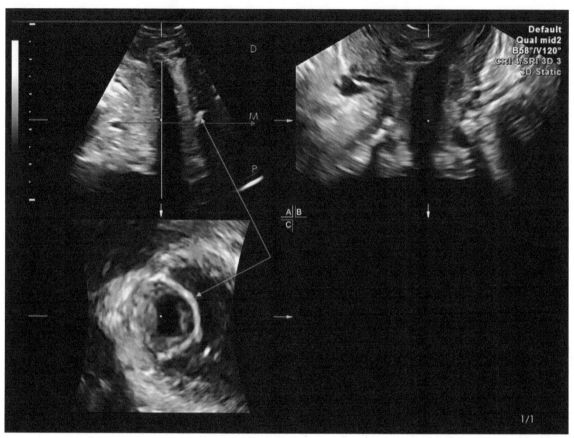

Fig. 381

CASE 177, FIGURE 382

22. Fig. 382 demonstrates four transperineal images of the ASC using a 6–12 MHz EV transducer with degrees of altered PRF to the Color Power Doppler. Identify which image is:

a. PRF that is too low _____

b. PRF that is acceptable _____
c. PRF that is too high _____
d. PRF that is the most appropriate _____

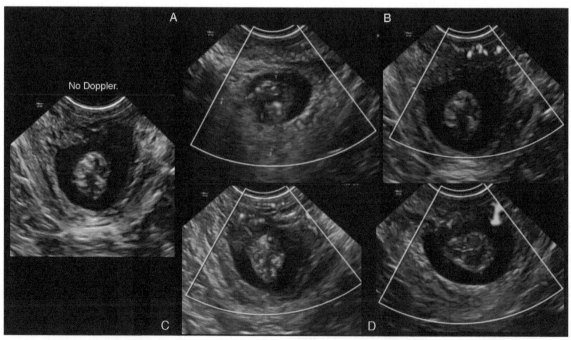

Fig. 382

CASE 178, FIGURE 383

23. Fig. 383 demonstrates a midsagittal image of the uterus on a postmenopausal 60-year-old woman. Which of the following is true about her endometrium?
    a. It measures normal at 2 mm and appears smooth in contour.
    b. It measures abnormal at 4 mm but appears smooth in contour.
    c. It measures abnormal at 2 mm and appears irregular in contour.
    d. It measures normal at 4 mm but appears irregular in contour.

24. Which of the following indicates a normal Color Power Doppler flow pattern of the endometrium?
    a. The arcuate arteries lie perpendicular to the endometrium at the uterine periphery and cross the myometrium.
    b. The radial arteries lie parallel to the endometrium within the intramural uterine segment.
    c. The spiral arteries lie perpendicular to the endometrium and do not cross the endometrium.
    d. The vascular pattern cannot be determined with Color Power Doppler.

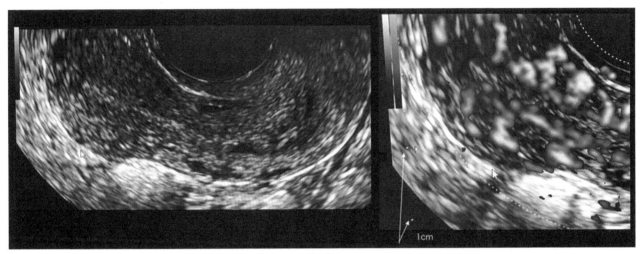

Fig. 383

CASE 179, FIGURE 384

25. Fig. 384 demonstrates transperineal ASC images of the A (sagittal) and B (transverse) planes of a 3D volume set. The patient is experiencing anal incontinence, and the clinician suspects a disrupted ASC and potential rectovaginal fistula. Which of the following statements is *not* true?
    a. There is a disruption of the mid-IAS at 1 OC with minimal elevation of the central mucosa toward the defect.
    b. The gold arrow is pointing to the tracking between the IAS and the posterior vaginal wall.
    c. The sagittal image demonstrates IAS disruption at the CRP that corresponds to the B plane CRP.
    d. The green arrow is pointing to the right pubovisceralis muscle complex.

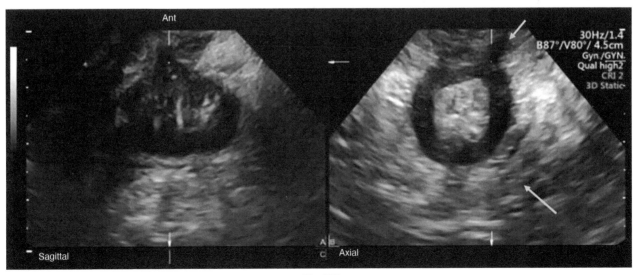

Fig. 384

CASE 180, FIGURES 385–389

26. Figs. 385–389 represent the pelvic anatomy of a 16-year-old patient whose last menstrual period was 6 days ago. She had an ultrasound exam a month ago at another imaging center. Today's exam is a follow-up to reassess a diagnosed pelvic mass. Because of her age and nonsexual activity status, all images were made using a 1–5 MHz curvilinear 2D transducer (more global information) and a 2–6 MHz transabdominal 3D transducer.

Fig. 385. 2D images of a normal left ovary (screen bottom) and the enlarged right ovary and the uterus (screen top) are shown. Remember, a normal ovary measures $1 \times 2 \times 3$ cm with a volume of about 3 cm³.

Fig. 387. What is the volume of her right ovary? _____

27. Based on the overall 2D and 3D images, which of the following best describes the right ovarian mass echo pattern?
   a. Round, poorly circumscribed hypoechoic lesion with enhanced through transmission (ETT)
   b. Round, complex, primarily solid-appearing lesion with diffuse luminal wall irregularity
   c. Oval, complex, primarily cystic-appearing lesion with ETT and irregular contour
   d. Oval, complex, primarily cystic-appearing lesion with focal mural wall thickening along posterior/right lateral luminal wall

28. Fig. 386 demonstrates a 3D volume set with rendered image of the mass with no changes of the green line of reference made (LOR), and Fig. 387 is another 3D volume set without the rendered image; therefore, no LOR is even on the image. When a 3D volume sweep is made, the CRP automatically becomes the center of the volume, no matter how wide the sweep is or in what plane the sweep is made. While the three orthogonal planes demonstrate the mass from different perspectives, this image is only the starting point to emphasize areas of concern when moving the CRP.

Fig. 388. By moving the CRP to the area of concern (gold arrow), all three orthogonal planes now demonstrate the irregular mural wall thickening. By bringing the LOR *to* the lesion on the "A" and "B" planes, the markedly abnormal luminal wall excrescences of the rendered image are appreciated on the rendered view (screen bottom right) and Fig. 389.

Answer the following.
a. The CRP is at the center of the Figs. 386 and 387 and has not been moved yet since the initial sweep location. If the "A" plane is *transverse* on Fig. 386, identify the direction of the green diamond icon on the "B" plane. _____
b. If the "A" plane is transverse on Fig. 386, identify the direction of the green square icon on the "B" (sagittal) plane. _____

Surgical pathology diagnosed a borderline tumor.

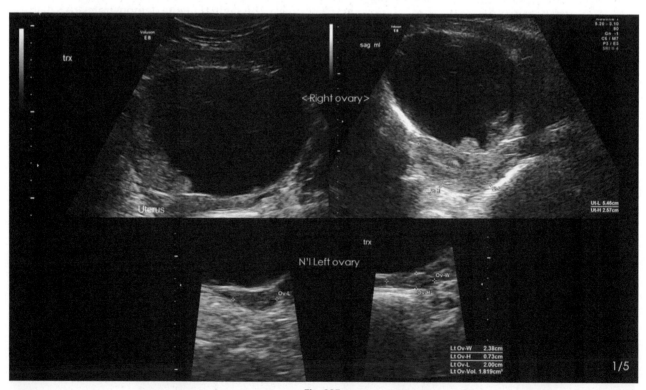

Fig. 385

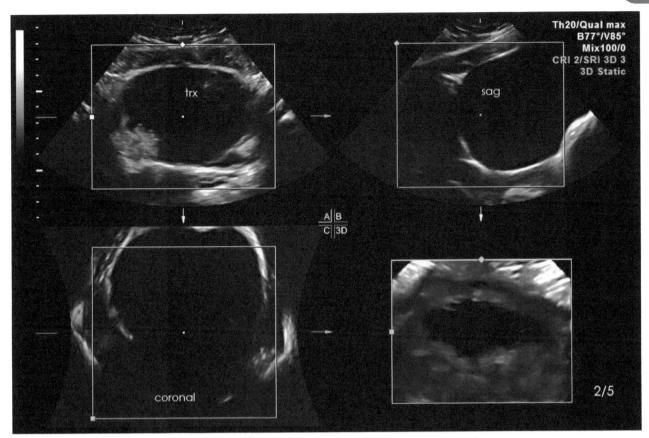

Fig. 386

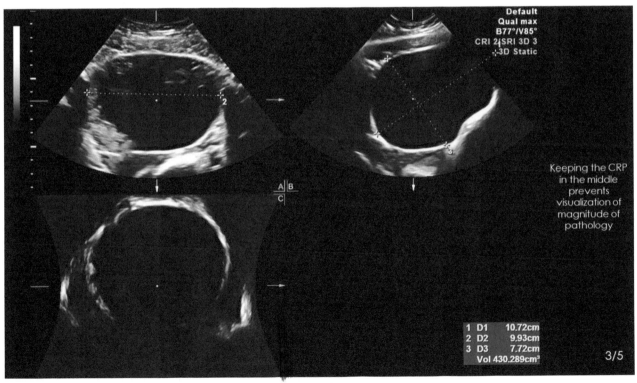

Fig. 387

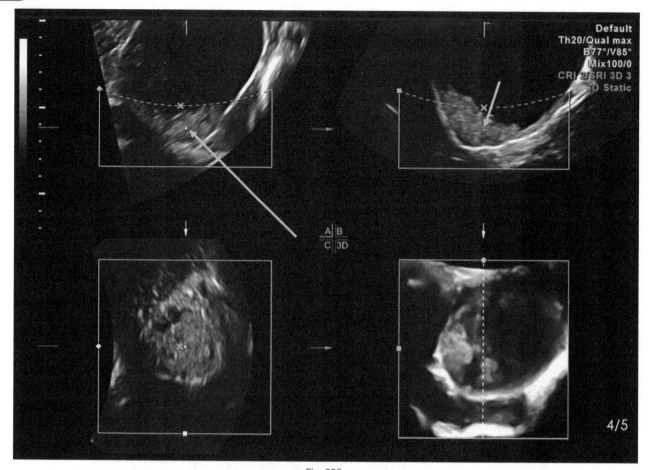

Fig. 388

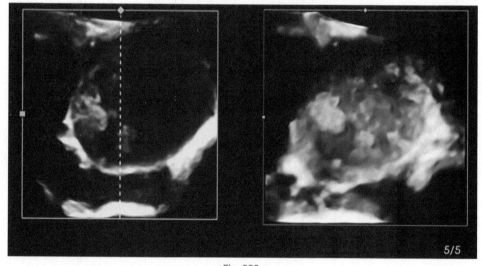

Fig. 389

CASE 181, FIGURES 390–395

29. Figs. 390–395 are images, using a 5–9 MHz EV transducer, of 30-year-old patient referred for pelvic pain and menometrorrhagia, or abnormal uterine bleeding (AUB), since delivery 10 weeks ago. A Mirena intrauterine device (IUD) was placed at her 6-week postpartum appointment. The left ovary appears within normal limits (WNL) and is not presented. The right ovary is seen on Fig. 391 (blue arrows) and appears WNL. In what position is the uterus—anteverted (AV), retroverted (RV), anteflexed (AF), or retroflexed (RF)?

a. RV

b. AV

c. RV, AF

d. AV, AF

e. RV, RF

30. Which two of the following describe the endometrial/myometrial interface appearance?
    a. Well differentiated with clear demarcation
    b. Poorly differentiated with indistinct demarcation
    c. Smooth in contour with homogeneous echo pattern
    d. Irregular in contour with homogeneous echo pattern
    e. Irregular in contour with heterogeneous echo pattern
31. Fig. 391. To what is the gold arrow pointing? _____
32. Fig. 391. Within the endometrium, there is an irregular globular hyperechoic area noted, measuring 2 × 2 cm, extending from the mid to the fundal aspect of the cavity (green arrows).

Figs. 392–394. Of note, all images demonstrate diffuse mottled uterine heterogeneity and increased uterine vascularity as well as increased endometrial vascularity as seen on 2D and Color Power Doppler (Fig. 392), which was thought to be consistent with myometritis.

Fig. 393 is a 3D volume set where the CRP is placed at the center of the volume. Note that the C plane (white arrow) demonstrates the arms of the IUD at the fundal portion of the endometrial cavity (gold arrow).

Figure 394 is a 3D volume set with rendered image where the CRP is seen to have been moved to the central lower uterine segment, which is best seen on the A plane (green arrow). Because the uterus is RV, the green square icon clarifies the right aspect of the uterus on the rendered image.

Fig. 395 demonstrates three images of a parallel shift through the upright uterine rendered image from the anterior to posterior endometrium. Which one of the following includes the correct multiple findings?
a. Abnormal IUD location, normal uterine echo and vascular pattern, retained products of conception, abnormal endometrium
b. Normal IUD location, abnormal uterine echo and vascular pattern, normal endometrium for 10 weeks postpartum
c. Abnormal IUD location, normal uterine echo and vascular pattern, retained products of conception
d. Normal IUD location, abnormal uterine echo and vascular pattern, retained products of conception, abnormal endometrium

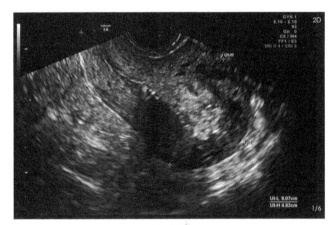

Fig. 390

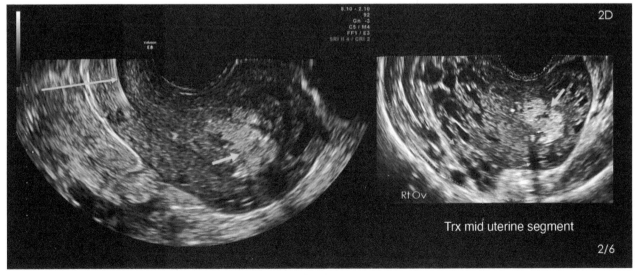

Fig. 391

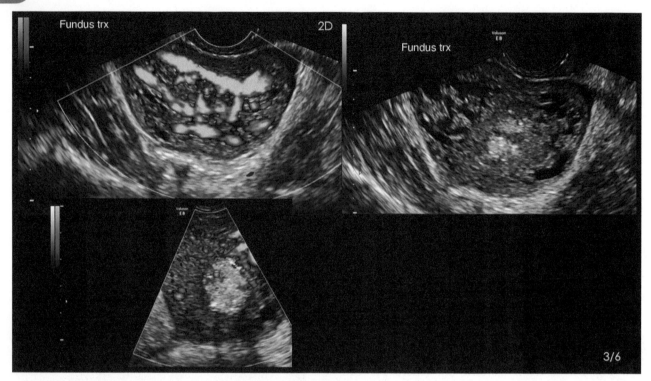

Fig. 392

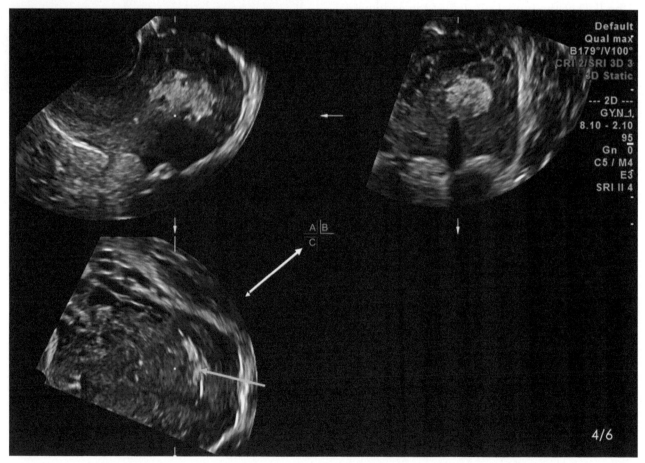

Fig. 393

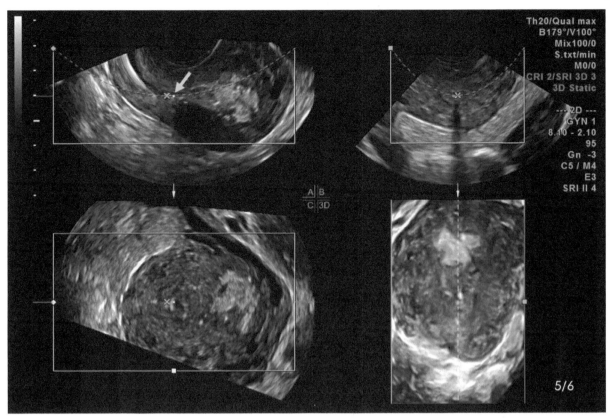

Fig. 394

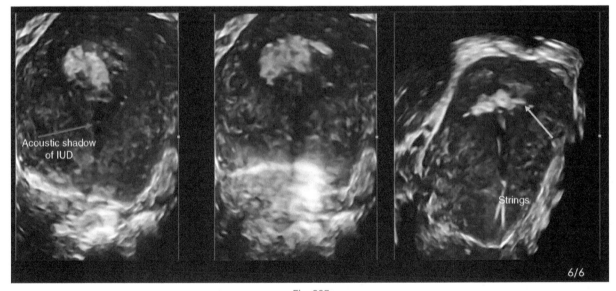

Fig. 395

CASE 182, FIGURE 396

33. Fig. 396. A 61-year-old patient was referred for an urogyn exam with a suspected rectocele. A transperineal exam was performed using a 6–12 MHz EV transducer. The 2D imaging demonstrated an unusual curved appearance of the IAS. By performing a 3D volume sweep of the ASC, the serpiginous appearing IAS of the A plane (white arrow) was traced with OMNI, which is like a custom trace drawn through a 3D volume to "stretch out" a specific structure that appears folded over itself, such as this IAS, in order to be confident that it is all one contiguous structure. Normally, the ASC is viewed longitudinally or transversely through sectional cuts, but the normal complex is not folded over itself. Remember, the IAS appears hypoechoic and the central mucosa appears hyperechoic. When the trace is then "stretched out" from quadrant A (screen right), is the IAS contiguous or not contiguous on quadrant 1 (gold arrow)?

_____

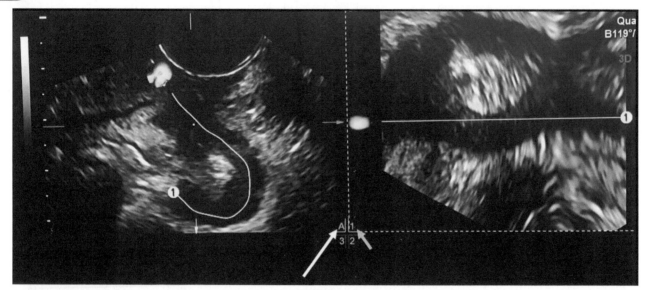

Fig. 396

CASE 183, FIGURE 397

34. Fig. 397 is a midsagittal EV image of a non-pregnant cervix using a 6–12 MHz EV transducer. Which of the following descriptors is incorrect?
   a. The cervix parenchyma appears diffusely homogeneous, which is abnormal.
   b. The cervical canal appears as a fine central curvilinear structure, WNL.
   c. There is trace-free fluid noted in the posterior cul-de-sac, which is WNL.
   d. Hyperechoic bowel is seen adjacent to the posterior cervical segment, which is WNL.

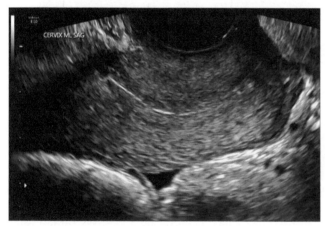

Fig. 397

CASE 184, FIGURE 398

35. Fig. 398 is a transperineal midline sagittal image of the urethra, using a 3–9 MHz EV transducer, on a 57-year-old patient who has dysuria and minimal post-void urinary leakage. Relative to the proximal urethra, in what directions on the patient is the abnormal oval-shaped structure labeled?
   a. Inferior
   b. Superior
   c. Posterior
   d. Anterior
   e. Left
   f. Right
36. Is the abnormality anechoic? _____
37. Is the echo pattern of the abnormality homogeneous or heterogeneous? _____
38. Is the abnormality enveloped by a thick capsule? _____
39. Which of the following is the most likely diagnosis for this appearance?
   a. Urethral abscess
   b. Anterior vaginal leiomyoma
   c. Urethral diverticulum
   d. Paraurethral cyst

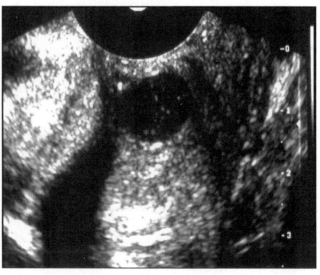

Fig. 398

Abbreviations

ACP, axis center point *aka* center reference point
AF, anteflexed
AI, anal incontinence
AP, anteroposterior
ASC, anal sphincter complex
AUB, abnormal uterine bleeding
AV, anteverted
BSO, bilateral salpingo-oophorectomy
c/w, consistent with
cc, cubic centimeter; cm^3; 1 cc = 1 mL
CRP, center reference point *aka* axis center point
DDx, differential diagnosis
DOV, depth of view
EAS, external anal sphincter
EDV, end-diastolic velocity
ETT, enhanced through transmission
EV, endovaginal
f/u, follow-up
FF, free fluid
FOV, field of view
FR, frame rate
Fr, French
hCG, human chorionic gonadotropin
IAS, internal anal sphincter
LLQ, left lower quadrant
LMP, last menstrual period
LOR, line of reference
LUS, lower uterine segment
MDV, mean diastolic velocity
MHz, megahertz
ML, midline
mL, milliliter; 1 mL = 1 cc

OC, o'clock
PAE, posterior acoustic enhancement
PAS, posterior acoustic shadow
PCDS, posterior cul-de-sac
PI, pulsatility index
PRF, pulse repetition frequency
PSV, peak systolic velocity
PVR, post-void residual
RF, retroflexed
RI, resistive index
RLQ, right lower quadrant
RV, retroverted
SUI, stress urinary incontinence
TAH, transabdominal hysterectomy
TGC, time-gain compensation
TOA, tubo-ovarian abscess
TOT, transobturator tape
TUI, tomographic ultrasound imaging
TVH, transvaginal hysterectomy
TVT, tension-free vaginal tape
WNL, within normal limits

2D, two-dimensional
3D, three-dimensional

mL, cm^3, and cc are used interchangeably
"transverse" and "axial" are used interchangeably
"cuts" and "planes" are used interchangeably
"midsagittal" and "ML sagittal" are used interchangeably
"transperineal" and "translabial" are used interchangeably
3D A, B, and C planes = 1, 2, and 3 planes

ASC NORMAL EXAM ASSESSMENT

Sonologist(s):

Findings:
A 2D transperineal exam, with the patient in the dorsal lithotomy position, was performed using a ___ 5–9 MHz *or* ___ 6–12 *or* ___ MHz EV transducer to assess the ASC and reveals a normal ASC, with measurements at three levels as follows:

Proximal level
The IAS measures ___ mm, ___ mm, ___ mm, and ___ mm at 12, 3, 6, and 9 OC positions.

Midlevel
The IAS measures ___ mm, ___ mm, ___ mm, and ___ mm at 12, 3, 6, and 9 OC positions.

Distal level
The IAS measures ___ mm, ___ mm, ___ mm, and ___ mm at 12, 3, 6, and 9 OC positions.

The EAS measures ___ mm, ___ mm, ___ mm, and ___ mm at 12, 3, 6, and 9 OC positions.

___ Color Power Doppler elicits normal ASC vascularity.
___ With pelvic floor contraction, there is normal shortening of the EAS.
___ 3D reconstruction confirms findings.
___ 3D volume transperineal assessment reveals normal PVM/pubic symphysis rami attachment with no evidence of PVM complex avulsion.

Additional comments:

ASC ABNORMAL EXAM ASSESSMENT

Sonologist(s):

Findings:
A 2D transperineal exam, with the patient in the dorsal lithotomy position, was performed using a ___ 5–9 MHz *or* ___ 6–12 MHz *or* ___ MHz EV transducer to assess the pelvic floor and reveals an **abnormal ASC**.

This is noted at the ___ proximal ___mid ___distal level(s), described with measurements as follows:

Proximal level
___ There is no disruption of the proximal IAS.
___ There is a disruption of the IAS from ___to ___ OC, with concomitant elevation of the central mucosa toward the defect. Color Power Doppler elicits ___ normal *or* ___ abnormal ASC vascularity.
The IAS measures ___ mm, ___ mm, ___ mm, and ___ mm at 12, 3, 6, and 9 OC positions.

Midlevel
___ There is no disruption of the mid-IAS.
___ There is a disruption of the IAS from___ to ___ OC, with concomitant elevation of the central mucosa toward the defect. Color Power Doppler elicits ___ normal *or* ___ abnormal ASC vascularity.
The IAS measures ___ mm, ___ mm, ___ mm, and ___ mm at 12, 3, 6, and 9 OC positions.

Distal level
___ There is no disruption of the distal **IAS**.
___ There is a disruption of the IAS from ___ to ___ OC, with concomitant elevation of the central mucosa toward the defect. Color Power Doppler elicits ___ normal *or* ___ abnormal ASC vascularity.
The **IAS** measures ___ mm, ___ mm, ___ mm, and ___ mm at 12, 3, 6, and 9 OC positions.

___ There is no disruption of the **EAS**.
___ There is disruption of the EAS noted from ___ to ___ OC. Color Power Doppler elicits ___ normal *or* ___ abnormal ASC vascularity.
The **EAS** measures___ mm, ___ mm, ___ mm, and ___ mm at 12, 3, 6, and 9 OC positions.

___ With pelvic floor contraction, there is normal shortening of the EAS.
or
___ The patient is unable to perform a pelvic floor contraction.

___ 3D reconstruction confirms findings.
___ 3D volume assessment reveals normal PVM/pubic symphysis rami attachment with no evidence of PVM complex avulsion.

or
___ 3D volume assessment of the pelvic floor reveals an asymmetric PVM complex. There appears to be an avulsion noted along the ___ left, ___ right, *or* ___ bilateral aspect of the vaginal wall, measuring approximately ___ cm.

Additional comments:

SONOHYSTEROGRAPHY ASSESSMENT

Sonologist(s):

Findings:
A sonohysterogram, with the patient in the dorsal lithotomy position, was performed using a ___ 5–9 MHz *or* ___ 6–12 MHz *or* ___ MHz EV transducer and reveals a(n) ___ anteverted ___ retroverted *or* ___ neutral uterus of normal size and contour.

___ The uterine echo pattern appears homogeneous, with no myomatous lesions identified.
or
___ There are several well-circumscribed myomatous lesions identified, the largest located at the _____ uterine segment *or other specific location*, measuring ___ cm, and located _____ relative to the endometrium. The echo pattern is heterogeneous with a decreased central echo pattern, suggesting some degree of degeneration. Color Power Doppler reveals a peripheral concentric flow pattern around lesion(s). Findings are c/w leiomyomata.

The endometrium is ___ heterogeneous *or* ___ homogeneous in echo pattern; ___ irregular *or* ___ smooth in contour, and measures ___ mm in AP diameter; *or* ___ ranges from ___ to ___ mm in AP diameter.

Both the ovaries are well visualized and appear WNL in size and echo pattern. Several follicles are seen bilaterally, appearing normal in size and number.

Under sterile conditions and with patient consent, a sonohysterogram was performed using a ___ 5-French Goldstein catheter *or* _____ catheter.
___ cc sterile saline was infused without incident.

Findings within the cavity include the following:
___ A single *or* ___ Several/Multiple endometrial lesion(s) measuring in size from ___ to ___ mm are visualized and appear ___ isoechoic compared with the adjacent endometrium. Color Power Doppler reveals feeder vessels entering centrally into the lesion(s). Findings are c/w endometrial polyps.
or

___ A single *or* ___ Several/Multiple lesions within the endometrial cavity are noted, ranging in size from ___ to ___ mm. The echo pattern of the lesions is isoechoic to myometrium and appears to originate at the _____ aspect of the myometrium. Color Power Doppler reveals peripheral concentric flow pattern of the lesions. Findings are c/w submucosal myoma.

Post procedure, ___ mL of free fluid is noted within the PCDS, indicating patency of at least one tube.
___ 3D reconstruction confirms findings.

Additional comments:

GYNECOLOGIC ABNORMAL EXAM ASSESSMENT

Sonologist(s):

Findings:
A transperineal exam, with the patient in the dorsal lithotomy position, was performed using a ___ 5–9 MHz *or* ___ 6–12 MHz *or* ___ MHz EV transducer to assess the pelvic anatomy and reveals a normal urethra, measuring ___ cm in length. The bladder/urethral neck AP diameter measures ___ mm, changing to ___ mm with cough. No urethral abnormality is noted.
or
___ The urethra appears abnormal, *describe.*

___ Transabdominal and ___ EV exam reveals a(n) ___ retroverted, ___ neutral ___anteverted uterus of normal size and contour.
There are several well-circumscribed myomatous lesions identified, the largest located at the _____ uterine segment(s), with measurements ranging in size from ___ to ___ cm. The lesion(s) are located _____ relative to the endometrium.
The echo pattern is heterogeneous with a decreased central echo pattern, suggesting some degree of degeneration.
Color Power Doppler reveals a peripheral concentric flow pattern around lesion(s). Findings are c/w leiomyomata.

The endometrium appears ___ smooth ___ irregular in contour.
___ There is a trilaminar appearance of the endometrium, c/w the proliferative phase of the endometrial cycle with the AP diameter measuring ___ mm. *or*
___ The endometrium appears homogeneous in echo pattern, c/w the secretory phase of the endometrial cycle with the AP diameter measuring ___ mm. *If abnormal, describe.*

Ovaries
Right: Well visualized. Contains follicles of normal size and number.
Size: WNL

Echo pattern: WNL
Left: Well visualized. Contains follicles of normal size and number.
Size: WNL
Echo pattern: WNL

If ovarian abnormality is present, describe in terms of echogenicity, size, contour, Color Flow pattern, and Doppler velocity.
___ There is negative FF within the PCDS.
___ There is FF present within the PCDS, the volume measuring ___ cm³.
(Obtain two planes of the maximum FF and multiply L x W x H x 0.52 to obtain volume, knowing that mid-cycle FF up to 10 mL is normal.)

___ The ASC appears WNL.
or
___ The ASC demonstrates a disruption from ___ to ___ OC at the ___ proximal ___ mid ___ distal IAS *and/or* ___ EAS with elevation of the central mucosa toward the defect. Color Power Doppler elicits hypervascularity within this area. Findings are c/w vaginal delivery history.

___ 3D reconstruction confirms findings.

Additional comments:

GYNECOLOGIC NORMAL EXAM ASSESSMENT

Sonologist(s):

Findings:
A transperineal exam, with the patient in the dorsal lithotomy position, was performed using a ___ 5–9 MHz *or* ___ 6–12 MHz *or* ___ MHz EV transducer to assess the pelvic anatomy and reveals a normal mobile urethra, measuring ___ cm in length. The bladder/urethra neck measures ___ mm, changing to ___ mm with cough. Good mobility of the urethral neck is noted.

___ Transabdominal *and/or* ___ EV exam reveals a(n) ___ anteverted ___ neutral ___ retroverted uterus of normal size (as documented from exam measurements) and normal contour. No myomatous lesions are identified. The cervix appears WNL with ___ normal *or* ___ absence of nabothian cysts noted.

___ The endometrium is smooth in contour and thin in AP diameter, measuring ___ mm. *or*
___ The endometrium appears trilaminar in echo pattern, measuring ___ mm in AP diameter; findings are c/w proliferative phase. *or*
___ The endometrium appears homogeneous in echo pattern, measuring ___ mm in AP diameter; findings are c/w secretory phase.

Both the ovaries are well visualized and appear WNL in size and echo pattern, as documented from exam measurements. Additionally, both the ovaries contain several follicles of normal size and number.
___ There is no FF noted within the PCDS.

___ The ASC appears WNL.
or
___ The ASC demonstrates a disruption of the ___ proximal ___ mid ___ distal IAS *and/or* EAS *level* from ___ to ___ OC, with elevation of the central mucosa. Color Power Doppler elicits ___ normal *or* ___ increased vascularity within this area. Findings are c/w vaginal delivery history.
___ 3D reconstruction confirms these findings.

Additional comments:

GYNECOLOGIC SURGICALLY ABSENT UTERUS ASSESSMENT

Sonologist(s):

Findings:
A transperineal exam, with the patient in the dorsal lithotomy position, was performed using a ___ 5–9 MHz *or* ___ 6–12 MHz *or* ___ MHz EV transducer to assess the urethra and reveals a length of ___ cm with normal mobility. The bladder/urethra neck AP diameter measures ___ mm, changing to ___ mm with cough. No urethra abnormality is noted.
or
The urethra appears abnormal, *describe.*

EV exam reveals a surgically absent uterus. The vaginal cuff appears smooth in contour and echo pattern.
or, if cervix is present
The cervix is well visualized and appears normal.
or
The cervix is well visualized and appears abnormal, *describe.*

Both the ovaries are well visualized and appear WNL in size and echo pattern. Follicles of normal size and number are seen bilaterally.
If one or both ovaries are abnormal, describe it in terms of echogenicity, size, contour, Color Flow pattern, and Doppler velocity.

There is no intraperitoneal FF noted.

___ The ASC appears WNL with no disruptions noted.
or
___ The ASC demonstrates a disruption from ___ to ___ OC at the ___ proximal ___ mid ___ distal IAS *and/or* ___ EAS, with elevation of the central mucosa toward the defect. Color Power Doppler elicits hypervascularity within this area. Findings are c/w vaginal delivery history.

___ 3D reconstruction confirms these findings.

Additional comments:

PELVIC FLOOR MESH ASSESSMENT

Sonologist(s):

Findings:
A transperineal exam, with the patient in the dorsal lithotomy position, was performed using a ___ 5–9 MHz *or* ___ 6–12 MHz *or* ___ MHz EV transducer to assess the urethra and bladder and reveals normal urethral contour and mobility. The urethral length measures ___ cm with AP neck diameter of ___ mm. With cough, the urethra demonstrates dynamic posterior movement and ___ opening *or* ___ closure of the neck, measuring ___mm.

___ There is no evidence of an outpouching of the distal urethra that would be c/w a urethral diverticulum.
___ There is a hypoechoic well-circumscribed urethral wall bulge extending ___ posteriorly *or* ___ laterally from the distal urethra, measuring ___ mm. This evidence of an outpouching of the distal urethra from the border is c/w a urethral diverticulum. Color Power Doppler elicits ___ normal ___ abnormal vascularity of the peri-urethral vasculature.

___ With Valsalva, support of the pelvic floor anatomy is maintained.
___ With Valsalva, support of the pelvic floor anatomy is not maintained, as evidenced by ___ posterior *or* ___ posterior/inferior bulging of the ___urethra ___ bladder ___ vagina *and/or* ___ small bowel (enterocele).

___2D midsagittal imaging demonstrates a smooth, curvilinear hyperechoic echo complex that represents the presence of *mesh* posterior to the **proximal urethra**, not the mid-urethra. *or*

___ 2D midline sagittal imaging demonstrates a smooth, curvilinear hyperechoic echo complex that represents the presence of *mesh* posterior to the **mid-urethra**, which is at the ideal location. *or*
___ 2D midline sagittal imaging demonstrates a smooth, curvilinear hyperechoic echo complex that represents the presence of *mesh* at the **distal urethra**, not the mid-urethra.

___ The mesh, relative to the urethra, is ___ mobile with cough *or* ___ is not mobile with cough.
___ With Valsalva, the mesh appears to ___ support *or* ___ not support the ___ urethra ___vagina *and/or* ___ bladder.

___ The mesh is seen as bilaterally symmetric with no bulking along either side. *or*
___ The mesh is seen as bilaterally asymmetric with the _____ side thicker than the right, measuring ___ cm, as compared to ___ cm.

The bladder contour appears normal with a pre-void volume of ___ mL, changing to post-void volume of ___ mL.
The bladder wall measures ___ mm, which is ___ normal ___ abnormal in thickness.
___ There are no bladder luminal wall trabeculations noted.
or
There are ___ focal *or* ___ diffuse bladder luminal wall trabeculations noted.

3D reconstruction confirms these findings.

Additional comments:

Answer Key

Chapter 1: Case Reviews 1–18

2. a. The top of the screen is inferior on the patient.
    b. The uterus is anteverted with the fundus directed anteriorly (screen left on Fig. 4).
    c. The uterus is neither anteflexed nor retroflexed.
3. a. The posterior segment, though superior relative to the transducer
    b. The anterior segment, though superior relative to the transducer. If the uterus was retroverted/retroflexed, the opposite segments would be at the top and bottom of the screen on the sagittal plane.
4. a. This is transperineal in a ML sagittal plane. The image is as if looking up the patient from the distal urethra, starting inferiorly. Therefore, the top of the screen is inferior. The bottom of the screen is superior. Screen left is anterior. Screen right is posterior.
    b. This is transperineal of a cut 90 degrees to the A plane (orthogonal to the A plane at the dot as if looking anteriorly from behind the urethra); therefore, the cut is coronal of the urethra. The top of the screen is inferior.
    c. This is transperineal of a cut coronal to the dot seen on the A plane, as if looking from one side of the urethra to the other (green line); therefore, the cut is a transverse cut of the urethra. Screen left is anterior. Screen right is posterior. Screen top is the patient's left. The bottom of the screen is the patient's right.
    d. Superior
    e. Superior
    f. Anterior
    g. Right
5. Because the mesh is posterior to the CRP location.
6. The transducer should be angled anteriorly toward the patient's head by bringing the handle down to bring the fundus into view of this anteverted uterus.
7. Though thin, there are distinct layers—the hyperechoic basal layer (a), the hypoechoic functional layer (b), and the hyperechoic central cavity (c)—created by the two apposing walls of the central cavity. Therefore, this demonstrates the early proliferative phase. The endometrium is often erroneously called a "stripe" but, because it changes by the day in appearance, that term should be removed from reporting descriptive terminology. There are other cases at other phases presented in this workbook.
8. The letter "d" is pointing to a loop of small bowel in cross-section (as if it is coming at you).
9. No. It should be moved up to the uterus level. This would improve the resolution of the anatomy at this level. Additionally, the depth of view for the image could be improved by decreasing the field of view, since half the screen is imaging bowel and our area of interest is the uterus.
10. The uterus is retroverted.
11. This is the anterior segment directed back posteriorly.
12. Inferior
13. Superior
14. Posterior
15. Anterior
16. The transducer should be angled posteriorly toward the patient's feet to bring the fundus into view of this retroverted uterus.
17. The endometrial segments are more obscured on this image. Though the functional component is now thickened, there remain three distinct layers—the outer hyperechoic basal layer (gold), the now thickened functional layer, isoechoic to the basal layer (green), and the hyperechoic central cavity (red)—created by the two apposing walls of the central cavity; therefore, this demonstrates the late secretory phase.
18. The CRP (red dot) on the B plane is placed on the left lateral echogenic focus; therefore, the A plane is sagittal at that left side with the white dot CRP corresponding to that same echogenic focus. The light blue dot CRP is the coronal cut through the uterus at that same level and the rendered image demonstrates the hyperechoic foci at the bilateral isthmus locations, proving the coil is correctly placed.
19. The perspective for this image is as if one is looking from posterior to anterior of the pelvic floor at a transverse cut of the urethra and mesh. The patient's right side is on the left of the screen.
20. c. Unless the entire volume set is present, the relative location of the mesh as compared to the urethral segments would not be known.
21. The mesh is located at the proximal urethra. Since the urethra is only 3–4 cm long and a small mesh placement difference can alter the effectiveness of the urethral/bladder function, the level should be reported on all cases.
22. A curvilinear, hyperechoic structure is visualized posterior and lateral to the urethra, consistent with history of former SPARC sling placement. Of note, the symmetric sling is located at the proximal (not mid) urethra in close proximity to the bladder neck.

    A small, round hyperechoic structure is seen in the posterior, proximal urethral wall on sagittal view, and is also visualized on coronal view and with 3D reconstruction. This does not change throughout the exam, suggesting the possibility of a foreign body such as a suture in the posterior urethral muscularis.
23. a. Myometrium
    b. IUD stem
    c. IUD strings
    d. Cornua

24. Measurements can be made using the calipers along the side of the images. The uterus is enlarged measuring 5.7 × 11.8 × 8.3 cm. The normal uterine volume changes throughout the menstrual cycle and ranges from 70 to 200 cm³. The formula to calculate volume is the prolate ellipsoid volume calculation, which is L × W × H × 0.52; therefore, the volume of this uterus is enlarged at 290.3 cm³.

25. b. The posterior/fundal myoma displaces the endometrium anteriorly giving the false impression of anteflexion.

26. c

27. d

28. c

29. a. 1. Inferior
     2. Left
     3. Superior
     4. Right
    b. 1. Inferior
     2. Posterior
     3. Superior
     4. Anterior

30. The most likely etiology of the complex primarily cystic appearing mass is a hemorrhagic follicular cyst with a dependent clot. While it looks large on the screen, it measures very small at 1.5 × 0.885 × 1.38 cm with a volume of 0.9526 cm³. The patient was re-examined 6 weeks later at which time it all had resolved.

31. a. 2.3 × 1.5 cm. This ovary appears within normal limits in size.
    b. 4.1 × 3.6 cm. This ovary appears enlarged.
    c. No. The right ovary has a normal echo pattern. The left ovary demonstrates a diffuse heterogeneous dense appearing echo pattern.

32. a. Yes, the ovarian contour is smooth.
    b. No, the contour is circumferentially irregular.

33. a. Normal small follicles are seen.
    b. There is a paucity of follicles seen.

34. Though there is a normal circumferential flow pattern around one small follicle, most of the ovary has inconsistent vascularity.

35. RI is an additional tool that when abnormally low, less than 0.4, may raise the index of suspicion for quickly forming hypervascularized tissue, such as a neoplasm. The RI in this case was high at 0.61, decreasing, but not eliminating, the concern for malignancy.

36. c. The right ovary was resected. At pathology, the sonographic bulky, enlarged, and dense area of the left ovary was found to be a dysgerminoma with corresponding abnormal vascularity.

37. The acquisition sweep was ML sagittal, as seen on the A plane.

38. The CRP is seen at the mid posterior vaginal wall.

39. The CRP could be moved to the screen left at mid-urethra on the A plane, which would move through the volume on the orthogonal B and C planes. Alternatively, the CRP could also be moved towards screen left on the C plane to the mid-urethra.

40. There is no evidence of avulsion, although there are several aspects of the volume set that would have improved visualization of the entire PVM complex had the following three instrumentation steps been taken. First, the A plane could have been rotated to the left on the screen by shifting the Z-axis knob. Second, the C plane screen right side could have been rotated upward also with the Z-axis knob to enhance symmetry of the 3D rendered image. Third, if the green line of reference was moved up on the screen (inferior on the body), it would have added the final aspect of the PVM attachment at the pubic rami.

41. a. The typical sonographic venous appearance is one of low visibility, generally measuring 1–2 mm. AP diameter > 5 mm is considered abnormal.
    b. Normal vessels likely increase in diameter with Valsalva and resume normal size at rest. Dilated venous structures with Valsalva may demonstrate increased AP diameter, as seen on Fig. 31, where the diameter (gold lines) measures 6.5 mm with Valsalva. This same increase in diameter may be accomplished when a patient has prolonged periods of standing up or heavy lifting.
    c. Pelvic Congestion Syndrome
    d. This appearance of diffusely dilated vessels is indicative of pelvic congestion syndrome, which has a prevalence of 39%. It is associated with an increasingly incompetent ovarian vein varices that results in reduced venous clearance and stasis. As the venous dilatation worsens, the vessels become diffusely tortuous as flow becomes retrograde. Patients may describe the fullness as if their "bottom is going to fall out" and occurs more frequently in multiparous patients for unclear reasons. The patient's chronic pelvic pain will usually reflect the degree of dilatation seen sonographically.

    When dilated, abnormal venous structures can be serpiginous in contour and unilateral or bilateral. Other imaging, including CT and MRI, also well visualize the altered dilated vasculature with this condition.

42. The uterus is anteverted.

43. b

44. Using the calipers along the side of the images, the smooth-walled central cavity lesion measures 4.3 × 1.8 × 2.5 cm.

45. Doppler Color Flow pattern is the key to the diagnosis. The transverse image demonstrates a single anterior feeder vessel entering centrally (Fig. 33), the finding c/w a large endometrial polyp as opposed to the typical peripheral vascularity of a myoma.

    The patient was undergoing evaluation for infertility, the polyp was resected, and the patient became pregnant 2 months later.

46. a. Endometrial lesions are found on all three cases, ranging from 3 to 40 mm, some originating from the anterior, some from the posterior, and some from both aspects of the endometrium.
    b. Fig. 35 demonstrates a single lesion seen on both planes.
    c. It demonstrates increased internal central, not peripheral, vascularity within each lesion.
    d. Yes. A thin basal layer is seen only, except the abnormal segments.
    e. No, the vascularity is a qualitative sample of vessel presence.
    f. Yes

47. c

48. Hydrosalpinx

49. The sweep plane (A) is midline sagittal.

50. e

Chapter 2: Case Reviews 19–35

2. The IAS disruption is from 9 to 1 OC, with elevation of the central mucosa toward the defect.

3. c

4. a. It is circumferentially smooth.
   b. Yes
   c. This is called "posterior acoustic enhancement," also known as "enhanced through transmission," indicating little absorption of sound as it traveled through the lesion by the increased echogenicity beyond the lesion.

5. a. The septae seen are variable in thickness.

6. It would be incorrect to call this lesion a "cyst." It is complex primarily solid in appearance with diffuse low-level echogenicity and multiple thick and thin septae noted.

7. b

8. a

9. a. Bladder
   b. Vagina
   c. Rectum
   d. Urethra

10. c. Best seen on the C plane.

11. a

12. It measures $5 \times 10 \times 10$ mm.

13. a. Both (red arrows)
   b. Small rectocele at the distal posterior vaginal/rectal interface
   c. Left pubovisceralis muscle complex

14. Neither image is right or wrong.

15. a. Endometrial functional layer
   b. Endometrial basal layer
   c. Central cavity wall
   d. Extra-uterine transverse cut of bowel loop

16. c

17. b

18. a. The uterus is anteverted.
   b. The uterine echo pattern is diffusely heterogeneous and appears unlike the normal uterus.

19. a

20. a. Typically, however, flow pattern of this condition appears randomly scattered.

21. c. It is not uncommon to find concomitant leiomyomata; however, no demonstrable myomatous lesions are seen in this patient.

22. Using the calipers along the side of the image, the transverse width measures 10 cm.
   a. The normal nulliparous uterine transverse width measures approximately 4–5 cm.
   b. i. The lesion is central in location, within the endometrial cavity.
      ii. The lesion is irregular and multilobular in contour.
      iii. The lesion is oblong and multilobular in shape, with the widest aspect at the transverse plane.
      iv. The echo pattern is complex primarily solid in echo pattern, with a rim of hypoechogenicity around most aspects of the mass, except the left lateral aspect where the lesion appears to be contiguous with the myometrium (gold arrows). All is thought to be within the endometrial cavity.

23. b

24. d

25. d

26. The volume measures 6.523 cm³ when calculated manually, which correlates with the volume on the image of 6.568 cm³ done at the time of the exam.

   This demonstrates that measurements can trustfully be calculated post exam using the prolate ellipsoid formula from two planes; therefore, one can measure the L × H × W × 0.52 to obtain the parameters and volume. This assumes one does not measure, say, the transverse width twice instead of the AP diameter; so, one must be sure what the directions are on each plane.

27. a and e. Describe the mass as anechoic, indicating it is simple, with a smooth though irregular border extending toward the patient's left side. The ultimate diagnosis requires histochemical assessment.

28. The volume of this ovary is measured on Fig. 56 and is markedly increased at 154 mL (cm³).

29. a. Smooth
   b. Bilobular
   c. Heterogeneous

30. Both and, cumulatively, markedly increased.

31. RI = 0.2

   The RI of this ovary is abnormal. Sometimes, a benign process changes flow patterns to have a low RI. A typical corpus luteum, for example, has a low RI as it develops quickly. A malignant lesion tends to quickly form new vessels also with a low RI; so, in the context of imaging, a first exam often elicits a referral for a repeat exam in the presence of a mass with a low RI.

   It is crucial to repeat the imaging exam in enough time for a potential corpus luteum to resorb. It is reasonable to schedule after 8 weeks or at least two full menstrual cycles. Rushing to repeat another exam prior to that time may result in continued concerning 2D findings, Color Power Doppler, and abnormal spectral waveform patterns.

   These findings persisted on repeat exam and she underwent surgical removal of the mass. The pathologic diagnosis for this lesion was a borderline tumor.

32. a. They are the right and left pubovisceralis muscle complex, which is most optimally seen at the midlevel.
   b. Screen left on a transverse cut is right on the patient, as if looking "up" the patient (from inferior to superior).
   c. It is widely disrupted from 8 to 2 OC (green arrows), with elevation of the central mucosa (CM) toward the defect.

33. 3.38×2.69 cm

34. More

35. 2D EV imaging of the IAS and perianal tissue demonstrates a disruption from 8 to 2 OC at the midlevel IAS, as seen by the presence of the pubovisceralis muscle complex posterior and lateral to the IAS. Anterior to the disruption is a poorly demarcated heterogeneous perianal soft tissue area with irregular contour, and a central area measuring approximately 3.4×2.69 cm. Multiple punctate echogenic foci are noted within this central soft tissue area. 2D Color Power Doppler elicits diffusely increased vascularity throughout this area. 3D volume render demonstrating profound accumulated increased vascularity (Fig. 65).

   Findings are c/w a perianal abscess extending from a severe IAS disruption and vaginal tear.

   Over the next 8 weeks, the patent was treated medically with various antibiotics and the abscess gradually reduced in size and the patient slowly improved.

36. b

37. Yes, the stem is central.

38. No. Though the stem is central (Fig. 67), the arm extends beyond the cavity into the left myometrium (Fig. 68).

39. It is at the mid IAS by demonstration of the adjacent pubovisceralis muscle (PVM) complex. All quadrants of the IAS are measured, demonstrating relative symmetry with the central mucosa.

40. a. Central mucosa (CM)
   b. Left pubovisceralis muscle (PVM) complex
   c. Internal anal sphincter (IAS)

41. Label E is the patient's right side and F is left as if you are looking inferiorly to superiorly.

42. No. The absence of the pubic and anterior/lateral PVM makes this diagnosis inconclusive. To be complete, another 3D volume sweep needs to be performed with an angulation of the line of interest from symphysis to the puborectalis level wide enough sweep angle to include all anatomy anteriorly to posteriorly. This is usually accomplished with the CRP moved to symphysis and the plane rotated on the Z-axis.

43. Appreciating the 90-degree planes' yin-yang appearance of an acutely formed hemorrhagic clot is related to knowing what direction is where on each plane of an EV image. When a clot forms, it lies at the dependent portion of the hemorrhage at the dependent portion of the patient in a layer/layer (fluid/fluid) pattern. So, if the patient is lying down, the dependent aspect is inferior (always at the top of the screen when the exam is EV). What is seen in the sagittal versus transverse plane is related to the side locations. In the sagittal plane, screen left is anterior (screen right posterior) and in the transverse plane, screen left is the right side of the patient (screen right is the left side of the patient).

   Fig. 72a is labeled with correct directions on the patient as related to each aspect of the clot of the sagittal and transverse plane.

44. a. Yes. The typical normal ovary measures $1 \times 2 \times 3$ cm with a volume of approximately 3.12 mL (cm³). Globally, this ovary measures 1.5×2 cm.
   b. The contour of the ovary is smooth in appearance; the hyperechoic subcomponent is eccentric yet also smooth in contour within the ovary.
   c. If her last menstrual period (LMP) was 1 week ago, her ovary would be in the follicular phase and demonstrate several small follicles. No follicles, normal or abnormal, are seen within the ovary on these cuts;

however, if a higher-frequency transducer could have been used, there may have been a few small follicles visualized.

45. a

46. Too high

47. c

48. It is not entirely visualized by transperineal imaging due to distal apposition of the mucosa and possible minimal transducer compression; however, the urethra appearance is typical.

49. This is an example of how important assessing anatomy in two planes is, especially in the presence of what may be perceived to be an abnormality. The finding is not uncommon in a partially full bladder.

50. a. Indistinct
   b. Endometrial periphery
   c. 16 mm
   d. 23 mm
   The endometrium appears thickened with a smooth contour and a relatively homogeneous echo pattern. The anteroposterior (AP) diameter measures 23 mm, whereas the typical measurement would be 5–7 mm at the early proliferative phase. The endometrial layers are indistinct with the isoechoic thin basal layer noted peripherally only at the lower endometrium. The basal layers are being measured by the calipers at 1.5 and 1.7 mm.

51. Focal peripheral vessels extend centrally into the endometrial mass.

52. c

53. a. The typical bladder wall thickness is 1.5–2.76 mm.
      When the bladder is distended, it should not measure more than 3 mm.
      When the bladder is empty, it should not measure more than 5 mm.
      This bladder thickness is abnormal, ranging 6.1–6.3 mm.
   b. The AP thickness at the arrow measures 8 mm.
      Etiologies for increased bladder wall thickness may include chronic UTI/ infectious cystitis, bladder outlet obstruction, neurogenic bladder, and cystitis from radiation or chemotherapy exposure, and others.

Chapter 3: Case Reviews 36–55

2. The transabdominal examination approach is infinitely variable with individualized angulation necessary

in order to optimize assessment of the uterus.

3. a. B, C, and D are EV images as evidenced by empty bladder, closer approach to the anatomy, and improved resolution. Image A is a transabdominal image.
   b. No. Image A demonstrates the measurement of the uterine length suboptimally, and the bladder is not full enough to completely see the uterine fundus. Unless the transducer lines of sight are perpendicular to the endometrium, it will not be optimally assessable even if the uterus is measurable.
   c. C. The cervical canal is well demarcated because the curvilinear transducer's lines of sight are hitting both interfaces perpendicularly.
   d. Correct answer is B, C, and D images. B is secretory phase, C is early proliferative phase, and D is secretory phase.

4. a. Angled anteriorly. Bring handle down.
   b. Move halfway out of the vagina and angle slightly anteriorly.
   c. Move out of the vagina and anteriorly from the vaginal introitus on the perineum to be directly in front of the urethra.
   d. Move out of vagina, angle perpendicularly [90 degrees to the anal sphincter complex (ASC)] on the vaginal posterior wall (yellow line) toward ASC (unless anorectal transducer is utilized).

5. a. Anteriorly, with the transducer toward the patient's head, handle down.
   b. Posteriorly, with the transducer toward the patient's feet, handle up.
   c. Post-menses; the two very thin hyperechoic basilar layers are apposing each other with no visible functional layers.
   d. Secretory; the functional and basilar layers are isoechoic, relative to each other, and slightly hyperechoic, relative to the myometrium.

6. a. It measures $10.9 \times 14.8 \times 14.3$ mm.
   b. Round
   c. It appears isoechoic to the vagina with several peripheral hyperechoic curvilinear echoes with and without posterior acoustic shadow. Isoechoic structures are difficult to see, so the calcifications can be helpful to get the

examiner on the right pathway toward locating lesions.

7. a. It is posterior.
   b. It is posterior and inferior.
8. The B plane, relative *to the patient's body*, is coronal through the center reference point (CRP), and the C plane is axial through the CRP.
9. It is not seen on the B plane because the coronal cut (90 degrees, or perpendicular, at the red line on the A plane) is posterior to the urethra.
10. 10×10 mm
11. d. Myomas can have a range of echogenicity and calcifications.
12. a. What to report: The bladder luminal wall contour is irregular and diffusely jagged in contour with markedly abnormal thickening, measuring 9.3 mm. Remember, the maximal wall thickness of a partially full bladder should be 5 mm or less.
13. Bladder
14. a. The caliper units along the right side of the Color Power Doppler of Fig. 92 are 0.5 cm increments, with every two lines measuring 1 cm units. The left (normal) labium (Fig. 90) measures $2.69 \times 1.43 \times 2.96$ cm with a volume of 5.48 cm^3. The right (swollen) labium (Fig. 92) measures approximately $3.5 \times 2.5 \times 2.25$ cm with a volume of 10.23 cm^3, calculated by using the prolate ellipsoid formula of (L × W × H × 0.523); therefore, one can confidently say that the right labium is about twice the size of normal.
    b. Diffuse. What to report: Color Power Doppler demonstrates a diffuse markedly increased pattern of flow of the enlarged right labium, indicating an extensive inflammatory process, especially as seen cumulatively on the profoundly increased vascularity of the 3D rendered images. Follow-up exams demonstrated gradual reduction of the hypervascularity with antibiotic treatment.
15. b. The surrounding posterior and lateral pubovisceralis muscle complex (Label C) is the adjacent mid-level internal anal sphincter (IAS) landmark.
16. a. Sagittal
    b. Transverse (axial) at the mid-internal anal sphincter (IAS) (see gold arrows at PVM complex on both A and B planes).
    c. Coronal

d. The CRP should be moved screen left on the A plane, which is proximal on the ASC, to just before the anal angle (red *).
17. Parallel. In this case, abnormal vessels can be clearly visualized in a parallel pattern anterior and posterior to the endometrium on the sagittal images (screen left, top, and bottom). When the transducer is turned 90 degrees to a transverse cut, those vessels can be seen entering into the central area of an endometrial lesion in the zoomed transverse plane (blue arrows, screen right, top, and bottom). This indicates a classic endometrial polyp appearance. The lesion is surrounded by a thin isoechoic post-menses basal layer component (gold arrow) of the endometrium on the transverse cut.
18. e
19. a. 11–12 o'clock (OC)
    b. 11–1 OC
20. Both. Note that the normally round central mucosa extends towards the defect on both images.
21. Though B demonstrates a portion of the PVM (gold arrow), the sector width during the exam was set wider for A (blue arrow).
22. It would be better. A higher-frequency transducer has higher resolution images.
23. b
24. a. Disruption is from 10 to 2 OC.
    b. There is an elevation of the central mucosa (CM) toward the defect.
    c. False. The perianal tissue is abnormally distorted and heterogeneous, suggesting the presence of scarred tissue.
25. a
26. e
27. a. Widens
    b. Both
    c. No
    d. No
    e. Yes
28. a. No.
    b. Inferiorly
    c. No. The bladder has an irregular bilobular bulky appearance that expands with Valsalva. It prolapses inferiorly. There is no evidence of enterocele.
29. A
30. a. Yes. It appears to extend through the cuff.
    b. It lies directly adjacent to the left ovary but is hard to tell if they are adhered on the initial

image. With manual lower pelvic compression, the two structures separated on real time.
31. a. Sagittal midline
    b. Transverse mid-uterus
    c. Coronal of uterine body
32. The A image is always the sweep plane, but what plane that is will be determined by the examiner in how they hold the transducer. Midsagittal is the standard cut for the sweep plane in uterine assessment and the typical sweep angle is about 75 degrees to capture the whole uterus with the slowest sweep speed setting to obtain the highest resolution. The center reference point (CRP) indicates the location at which the B plane is cut at 90 degrees, or perpendicular (transverse cut) to the A plane, and C plane is coronal to the A plane and a coronal cut of the uterus.
33. The C plane is the only view that shows the entire IUD in this case. Since the coronal C plane is not seen on the 2D vaginal approach, unless the uterus is in a neutral position, seeing the entire IUD on one plane may not be possible.
34. The coronal C plane is most reliable *if* the original sweep plane is midline sagittal.
35. It is pointing to a commonly seen nabothian cyst.
36. No. Only the stem is within the cavity. Note that the left arm is extending into the left portion of the myometrium. Only identifying the presence of the stem will often miss this diagnosis.
37. Posterior
38. Each horizontal-to-horizontal distance caliper along the side of each image is 1 cm. Each horizontal-to-dot distance is 0.5 cm. The left ovary is enlarged, measuring $4.2 \times 4.2 \times 4.3$ cm using the markers on the side of each image, with a volume of 40.38 cm^3 (using the prolate ellipsoid volume formula of L × W × H × 0.52. This was acquired from the calipers along the image of the 3D volume set. Remember, normal ovarian measurements should be around $1 \times 2 \times 3$ cm with a volume of 3 cm^3.
39. c. The only anechoic components of this ovary are a few peripheral follicles. Otherwise, the ovary demonstrates diffuse low to midlevel echoes, a thick partial vertical septum, and a solid round component

at the inferior aspect of the abnormal appearing ovary.

40. All three RIs are abnormally low at 0.20, 0.22, and 0.26. Remember, normal RI for the ovary should be above 0.4. Added concern is raised for malignancy when septae demonstrate increased vascularity, as is seen here. At surgical pathology, this mass was found to be a borderline tumor.

41. Each line-to-dot distance is 0.5 cm; so, one can appreciate the distance of the mesh from the perineum at about 1.5 cm. The purpose of this image and cine loop is to demonstrate how mesh can be well seen with a high-frequency transducer. To determine the location of the mesh, relative to the urethra would be better presented with a 3D volume set; however, it is evident that the surgical mesh placement is too distal.

Chapter 4: Case Reviews 56–74

2. a. It measures 3.75 cm (green lines), which is normal, as the average urethra is 4 cm. Remember, that is only 1.5 inches, but with the standard small field of view, it always looks much larger than it really is.
   b. It measures 7.5 mm.
   c. The arrow is pointing to the nearly empty bladder (superior to the urethral neck).

3. The AP measurement is reduced to 4 mm (B) from the original measurement of 7.1 mm (A) at rest.

4. a. Yes
   b. Yes

5. Midlevel

6. Yes (gold lines)

7. b. The uterine wall is symmetric in appearance at the screen top. The measurements of the 12, 3, 6, and 9 OC aspects of the IAS appear symmetric. The focal zone indicator is hard to see as it overlies increased echoes of the anatomy behind it, but it is at the level of the puborectalis muscle (green arrow) posterior to the IAS.

8. 2 is the level seen on the C plane image, which is *not* the IUD, but instead, the acoustic shadow created by the absorbing high-density IUD. One would have to parallel shift the plane or move the CRP (green arrow) on the volume set to the IUD stem to see the actual IUD and not the acoustic shadow.

9. Approximately 5 mm

10. Each of the caliper segments is 0.5 cm; therefore, the distance from the transducer to the rectum is 2.1 cm. Though the perianal tissue is less than 1 inch in distance in this case, it is highly abnormal to be this swollen, distorted, and heterogeneous and should be reported in detail.

11. a. Fig. 129. Gold arrows surround the EAS, which is at the same level as the distal IAS.
    b. Fig. 130. The mid IAS is located at the surrounding PVM complex (blue arrows).

12. What to report: There are multiple findings.
    a. There is an irregular oval-shaped poorly circumscribed heterogeneous area visualized between the poorly distinguished posterior vaginal wall (screen top) and the anterior segment of the rectum.
    b. It measures 4 × 2.2 cm.
    c. The echo pattern is complex primarily solid in appearance.
    d. Color Power Doppler elicits marked diffuse hypervascularity, especially within the central component of the area.
    Fig. 129, located at the EAS level, demonstrates an intact sphincter at this level. Fig. 130, however, which is located at the mid IAS, demonstrates an IAS disruption at 10 OC and a second disruption with a hypoechoic tracking at 12 OC, both with elevation of the central mucosa (CM) (labeled white arrows on Fig. 131). Findings are consistent with a perianal abscess, IAS disruptions, elevation of the CM, and a developing partial rectovaginal fistula directly anterior to IAS disruption at 12 OC.

13. a. Yes. There is an IUD present within the central cavity. The IUD arms were seen within the endometrial cavity though not presented here.
    b. Yes. The line of reference was brought down to the area of interest on the A and B planes, which was directly above the stem.
    c. It is at the left lower uterine segment (LUS). This can be double checked by noting that plane B (transverse cut) has a small on-screen green box icon, which on any (correctly done) uterine transverse cut would be at the

patient's right side (gold arrow). The 3D rendered image (bottom right) displays that same green box icon on the same side as the B plane green box; therefore, it is also the patient's right. While the examiner usually knows what direction is where on the volume set and rendered images, when pathology is complicated, it is not so intuitive and use of the icons helps tremendously to confirm location.

14. Fig. 133 demonstrates the location of the protruding IUD through the back wall of the uterus to the anterior edge of the adjacent hypoechoic bowel wall. When looking closely, during and post exam, the CRPs (green arrows) are *on* the structure to where it was moved from the initial volume center. You might have to get out a magnifying glass to see them! On the A plane, the CRP color is white; on the B plane, it is red; and on the C plane, it is light blue (green arrows). There is an additional way to notice the intersection points of the CRPs. Note that wherever there is a CRP, there are two short lines, one arrowed, along the periphery of the plane cuts. If you connect the two sides of those lines, they go straight across the image and intersect the CRP.

15. The IUD hyperechoic structure, seen as if it is coming toward the viewer on the B plane, is the transverse plane and the CRP color on it is red (green arrow, magnified on zoomed image below); therefore, number "1" is the IUD and the hyperechoic interface numbered "2" is lateral (as are all those other horizontal linear echoes) that likely represents adjacent myometrial and vascular wall interfaces. Fig. 134 demonstrates partial invasion of the IUD into the adjacent bowel wall. Knowing exactly where the second IUD was located allowed the provider to remove it from the bowel wall without incident, which resulted in immediate relief by the patient.

16. The anterior posterior (AP) thickness measures 24.13 mm (red arrow), far exceeding a typical early proliferative stage thickness of the endometrium. The normal endometrial thickness at this stage

should be 5–7 mm. The thin basal layer is seen as a thin hyperechoic outer rim of the endometrial complex (Fig. 135, gold arrows).

17. b

18. d. The basal layer is very thin (gold arrows) and envelops an isoechoic thickened multilobulated complex that appears primarily solid, not a hypoechoic layer.

19. a. The typical polyp is isoechoic to the endometrial basal layer and hyperechoic relative to the myometrium.

20. With the CRP moved to this area on all three planes, it indeed suggests a well-circumscribed, round hyperechoic structure measuring 8 mm at the right LUS/cervical interface. The B and C planes of Fig. 137, however, demonstrate that between the transducer and this "lesion" is a normal anechoic nabothian cyst, behind which is a distinct area of enhanced through transmission, which would be present posterior to any anechoic structure and appear round on the axial cut. With a Z-axis rotation of the 3D rendered image (Fig. 138), it looks very real. In fact, however, it is an artifact. Additionally, there is a similar appearance inferiorly of another nabothian cyst. (Fig. 137, green arrows)

21. d

22. It is ML, as seen on the CRP placement of B and C planes.

23. b. It should be reported that the distance from the anechoic midline structure to the anterior LUS wall (Fig. 140, green line) measures 5 mm. As a cautionary description, in the event of a subsequent pregnancy, this may put the patient at an increased risk for complications, including uterine rupture or placenta acreta.

24. c. Using calipers alongside the image, uterine length measures 6.4 cm and the AP diameter measures 2 cm, both within normal limits for age. The endometrial thickness is thin, as expected, measuring 2 mm. The spiral artery pattern is typically perpendicular to the endometrial interface but should not enter the endometrium. Fig. 142a demonstrates an abnormal segment of vascularity with a segment crossing the endometrium (green arrow). Though the arrow points to what appears to be abnormal flow across the endometrium, the

presumed vessel could not be reproduced and is most likely a flash artifact. Given her age, an endometrial biopsy was performed which was normal. The etiology of her spotting was presumed to be related to pessary use.

25. Yes. Though both stems are present and central within the cavity, they appear very near the cervix (gold arrows), so our recommendation was to follow-up within 3 months to confirm their location. The patient did not return for follow-up.

26. b

27. d

28. a. No. Normal follicles are not seen, but this is only one slice of the ovary and normal follicles may very well be seen in other planes.

b. No, the free fluid is minimal (green arrow).

c. No, there are diffuse low echoes levels noted; therefore, nothing within the ovary is anechoic (without echoes).

d. Yes, suggesting the presence of blood in various stages of resolution (red arrows).

e. No, there is "posterior acoustic enhancement" present, which is a misnomer.

A better descriptor for this appearance would be "enhanced through transmission." The mechanism for this appearance is that the blood within the hemorrhagic cyst does not absorb sound like a solid mass or even normal tissue would; therefore, with the expected automatic near to far field time gain compensation (TGC) increase, the area beyond the cyst appears increased in echogenicity rather than the same, which normal tissue would demonstrate. In this case, though it looks posterior to the ovary, this enhancement is superior to the hemorrhagic corpus luteum on the screen, as the transducer is located inferiorly (at the top of the screen). Enhanced through transmission (arrows) beyond a hemorrhagic corpus luteum is a typical finding of an acute bleed and should be noted in the report as it is sonographic criteria for this finding.

29. No. It is related to the ever-important location of the center reference point (CRP) on the volume set

and not to any pathology at this area. Fig. 148 exemplifies the cuts through the CRP location for each orthogonal plane. The yellow line is the B plane and the green line is the C plane relative to the A plane. The red arrow points to the C plane coronal cut (green line). Note that the straight green line lies above the more curved endometrial/lower uterine segment, which, therefore, would not be seen on the C plane. Instead, the C plane would demonstrate the more hypoechoic myometrium above that central location.

30. Because the CRP perpendicular cut of the transverse B plane is more fundal on the endometrium, as depicted on the A and C center reference points (CRPs). Remember, the colored dots *are* the CRPs, and are all the exact same point on different planes; however, the A and B planes include adjacent anatomy beyond that CRP, but the B plane, which is perpendicular to the A plane at the intersection of the A and B planes, only demonstrates the transverse fundal cut, not the LUS.

31. The gold arrow is pointing to the bladder (nearly empty).

32. b

33. Fig. 151. The screen right "stretched out" cavity length measures 13.2 cm. Adding the 1.5 cm thickness of each myometrial outer rim now makes the total length of the uterus 16.2 cm. The A plane (Fig. 152) measurement of the uterus length at approximately 11.2 cm (green line) is 5 cm shorter than a traced length of the curved uterus on Fig. 151. The other uterine dimensions measured on this volume set include the yellow line measuring the uterine anterior posterior (AP) diameter at 7 cm (sagittal image) and the red line measuring the uterine width at 6.3 cm (transverse); therefore, the uterine volume of 371.5 cm³ on this patient, calculated using the prolate ellipsoid volume formula, far exceeds a normal nulliparous uterine volume, even with the shorter length used.

34. d. Though the endometrial cavity is hypoechoic relative to the surrounding myometrium, the echo pattern is complex with diffuse small linear echogenic foci. The vagina is normal in appearance and contains no fluid. Findings are

consistent with hematometra, an insidious accumulation of long-term menses obstructed at a closed cervix.

35. b. The endometrium is not definitively seen, so cannot be measured. The uterine length and AP diameter are on Fig. 152. The transverse mid-uterus image is not presented here; however, it measures 5.6 cm in width, which would make the volume of her uterus 153.8 cm³, which is more than twice the typical normal uterine volume. The echo pattern is diffusely bulky in appearance with a circumferentially irregular contour. It is heterogeneous though no definitive myomata are appreciated. The echo pattern relationship of the hyperechoic uterus relative to the hypoechoic cervix is abnormal. They should appear relatively isoechoic.

36. a. What to report about the cervix: The cervix demonstrates irregular contour with markedly abnormal punctate echogenic foci seen at the anterior inferior focal area of the mass (small light green arrows). Color Power Doppler (Fig. 154) demonstrates diffuse increased vascularity of the cervix. The Doppler spectral waveform RI (Fig. 155) is abnormal at 0.39 using a 0.40 cut-off threshold for neoangeogenesis. Even though the RI is just under 0.40, it would be considered abnormal. Findings are consistent with her clinically diagnosed cervical carcinoma.

37. a. Left
    b. Contiguous
    c. No. There is a second circular 3.5-cm hypoechoic lower uterine segment (LUS) myomatous lesion (labeled as number 2).
    d. Yes, there is a trace amount of FF present (white arrow).
    e. Yes, but only at the mid to fundus endometrium. The inferior aspect of the endometrium is obscured by the LUS myoma (number 2).

38. a

39. a. 1.8 cm
    b. Color Power Doppler demonstrates minimal peripheral flow. There is no intralesion flow present. The patient remains clinically asymptomatic and desires continued surveillance of the cyst.
    c. Calcific infiltrates can suggest some degree of chronic inflammation or a complex lesion.

Chapter 5: Case Reviews 75–94

2. a. #2
   d. #1
   f. #4
   i. #3

3. a. Mid-urethra
   b. Midsagittal
   c. Coronal
   d. Axial

4. a. 5
   b. 1
   c. 3
   d. 2
   e. 4

5. (Left image, Right image)
   a. Yes, Yes
   b. Yes, Yes
   c. No, No
   d. Yes, No
   e. No, Yes
   f. Yes, Yes

6. a. Yes
   b. No
   c. No
   d. Yes, though it is displaced by the presence of a thickened mesh
   e. Yes, on the right (yellow arrow)
   f. No
   g. No
   h. Yes

7. c. It is easy to think that all ASC images are the same until many separate exams are lined up to assess, at which time, it becomes apparent that there are many differences noted if one looks systematically. If there is a defect, the examiner can measure across it to gauge its size. The following cases are all separate individuals.

8. a. Distal IAS/EAS
   b. Yes
   c. N/A
   d. N/A
   e. Yes
   f. N/A
   g. No

9. a. Mid IAS
   b. No
   c. 9–2 OC
   d. Yes
   e. No
   f. Limited view
   g. No

10. a. Mid IAS
    b. No
    c. 11–1 OC
    d. Yes
    e. No
    f. Limited view
    g. No
    h. Color Power Doppler demonstrates hypervascularity of the right IAS/vaginal interface

from 11-12 OC, suggesting history of inflammation at this past disruption.

11. a. Mid IAS
    b. Yes
    c. No disruption
    d. No shift
    e. Yes
    f. Limited view
    g. No
    h. Increased vascularity along the right lateral IAS suggesting post-inflammatory healing

12. a. Mid IAS
    b. No
    c. 11–1, 4–8 OC
    d. Yes
    e. No
    f. No
    g. No

13. a. Distal IAS/EAS
    b. No. Both IAS and ES disrupted
    c. IAS 10–1 OC (calipers); EAS 11–1 OC (yellow arrows)
    d. Yes
    e. No
    f. N/A
    g. No

14. a. Distal IAS/EAS
    b. Yes
    c. N/A
    d. N/A
    e. Yes
    f. N/A
    g. No

15. a. Mid IAS
    b. Yes
    c. N/A
    d. No
    e. Yes
    f. Yes
    g. No

16. a. Mid IAS
    b. No
    c. 11–1 OC
    d. Yes
    e. No
    f. Limited view
    g. No

17. a. Distal IAS/EAS
    b. Yes
    c. N/A
    d. N/A
    e. Yes
    f. N/A
    g. No

18. It is not visualized because the CRP is placed at the posterior vaginal wall/rectal interface and the urethra is anterior to this level.

19. No, the IAS is disrupted from 10 to 1 OC with elevation of the central mucosa toward the defect (gold arrows).

20. The PVR, calculated by the prolate ellipsoid volume formula of $L \times W \times H \times 0.52$, is typically < 100 cc; therefore, the volume of 357.7 cc on the screen is markedly increased.

21. It appears smooth but bulky in contour.

22. c. No distal portion of the urethra was visible throughout the exam, even with only the slightest pressure on the perineum. While the urethral wall thickness is typically not measured, it would range from 2 mm to 5 mm when measured from the mucosal edge to the outer urethral wall; so, the thickness of this patient's urethral wall is diffusely increased at up to 7 mm with abrupt loss of visualization of the hypoechoic distal mucosa.

23. It appears diffusely jagged in contour with broad irregularity.

24. It is at the central aspect of the distal urethra.

25. c

26. Yes, the PVM complex appears symmetric bilaterally.

27. The vaginal contour appears within normal limits and does not suggest the presence of avulsion.

28. It is at the distal level. Note the 3D rendered image of Fig. 184. Out of context (axial cut), it appears as a normal suburethral sling in appearance; however, it is so distal at only 2 mm from the perineal surface that it provides no support.

29. Inferior (as indicated on transverse cut)/Posterior (as indicated on sagittal cut). Remember, if the transducer is at the perineum, the top of the screen is always inferior.

30. No

31. It is irregular in contour

32. Yes (Fig. 185, yellow *)

33. d

34. a. Sagittal
    b. Axial (transverse)
    c. Coronal

35. Yes, but barely. There is a sliver of the puboviceralis muscle (PVM) complex on that level (blue arrow).

36. 11–1 OC

37. Yes. It is mildly elongated anteriorly toward the defect on all axial cuts.

38. Yes. The hypoechoic disruption of the anterior IAS becomes more elongated as it extends toward the left aspect of the posterior vaginal wall (blue arrows).

39. Original. It is directly suburethral as seen on Fig. 190 (gold arrow).

The green arrow points to the second mesh.

40. a

41. The examiner can parallel shift through the green volume box to see anatomy at any level. This can be done during the exam or post exam to fine-tune anatomic assessment.

42. a

43. a. A
    b. C
    c. B
    d. E
    e. D

44. d. The complex appearance and mixed echogenicity of the lesion was consistent with a purulent urethral diverticulum at surgery.

45. a. E
    b. B
    c. A
    d. D
    e. C

The ultrasound exam revealed the presence of anterior vaginal mesh, as well as 2 suburethral slings. See yellow and blue arrows on the midsagittal view, as well as additional oblique views at screen right. Dynamic imaging demonstrated that she had a non-relaxing pelvic floor. The patient was taken to surgery where two separate slings were removed, in addition to anterior vaginal mesh.

46. IAS

47. EAS

48. EAS

49. 11–1 OC

Chapter 6: Case Reviews 95–111

2. a. Arcuate
   b. Radial
   c. Spiral

3. d. Vessels parallel to the endometrium are never normal, especially in the presence of what appears to be an elongated homogenous endometrial lesion, as seen here.

4. d. Branching of vessels parallel to the endometrium entering centrally into the cavity is never normal.

5. a

6. d

7. d

8. a. Inferior
   b. Posterior
   c. Superior
   d. Anterior

9. d

10. It is at the distal location at only 2-4mm from her perineum.

11. c

12. b

13. c

14. Fig. 210a is the same image as Fig. 210, now labeled correctly. With the transducer in place, it compresses the vagina from below, while the bilaterally large complex primarily cystic structure is approaching it from above. Remember, when using an EV transducer "superior" is at the bottom of the screen. Labeled directions are as follows:
    a. Inferior
    b. Posterior
    c. Superior
    d. Anterior

15. c

16. b

17. a. Sagittal
    b. Transverse, Coronal
    c. 3D rendered image
    The sweep plane of any 3D volume set is always the A plane.

18. a. Figure 218 demonstrates * (functional layer) and ^(basal layer)

19. b

20. d

21. c. Though it is centrally located posterior to the urethra (suburethral), one cannot tell out of context if it is at the mid-urethra level from a single transverse (axial) cut. Only the midsagittal plane demonstrates where the sling is relative to the proximal, mid, or distal levels. Of note, the sling is partially folded over itself at the mid portion of the mesh, not an uncommon finding.

22. c

23. b

24. a. Transverse
    b. Sagittal
    c. Coronal

25. c. The RV uterus (Plane 2) demonstrates a smooth fundus with no invagination of the outer contour. The two endometrial cavities are distinct above a single LUS endometrial cavity (gold arrow).

26. a. There is posterior cul-de-sac free fluid present, which should be noted was not present prior to the procedure.

27. Statements a and c are not true.

28. c

29. b

30. a. No, it appears asymmetric.
    b. No, there is a disruption of the anterior IAS contour at 1 OC that extends toward the posterior vaginal wall (where the transducer is placed).

c. Yes, it is directed toward the disrupted anterior left aspect of the IAS.

d. Yes, there is a broad elevation of the anterior IAS border.

e. Yes, there is only a small area of hypoechogenicity where the CRP lies on the extended disruption. Findings are consistent with a developing rectovaginal fistula of unknown origin.

31. c. Though the typical nabothian cyst measures 2–10 mm, the normal range is quite variable and may be as large as 4 cm.

32. The typical uterine volume measures 75–200 cm³.

33. b, e, and g

34. b. There is profound uterine vascularity noted along the anterior aspect of the mass with focal peripheral flow extending to the anterior aspect of the mass. Minimal intramass flow is seen. 3D rendering confirms this appearance.

35. b. This is determined by review of the 3D volume set (Fig. 235) where the B plane, which is transverse, demonstrates the green square directional icon on the right side (red arrow). Of note, the green diamond icon (blue arrow) is located anteriorly on the A (sweep) plane, confirming the anterior location on the 3D rendered image.

36. a. Smaller. It now measures 5.3 cm.
    b. Irregular
    c. Oblong
    d. More heterogeneous
    e. Decreased peripheral vascularity

37. c. Though the patient was asymptomatic, she elected to have a hysterectomy, which was pathologically found to, indeed, be a degenerating leiomyoma.

Chapter 7: Case Reviews 112–128

2. a–d. Since it is subjective, any answer comparing the left image with the right image is correct.

3. c

4. The CRP is seen (gold arrows); however, the mesh is not seen at this level because the residual mesh is located elsewhere, which may be above the green curved line of reference on Fig. 241, which is inferior on the patient, toward the top of the screen.

5. Yes, it is seen. The gold arrow points to the subtle partial segments of mesh seen in all planes.

6. e

7. All aspects of this description are correct, except d; the tracking (gold arrows, Fig. 246) is directed toward the patient's left, not the right.

8. b

9. d

10. a. Yes, it appears symmetric.
    b. There is no evidence of an avulsion.
    c. Yes, it is symmetric.

11. The correct answer is B with noted bilateral lateral vaginal wall bulging. Avulsion is damage to the pubovisceralis muscle complex related to detachment of the muscle from its insertion on the inferior pubis rami with overstretching of the levator muscle complex during the second stage of labor. The prevalence may be up to 36% of all first-time deliveries, reducing drastically to 0.9% with the second delivery. As a result, there is hiatal ballooning and subsequent issues with pelvic organ prolapse and/or anal incontinence.

12. a. True
    b. True
    c. True. This is evidenced by the posterior/inferior displacement of the bulging bladder/urethral neck interface.
    d. Not true. Even though it is nearly empty, the bladder bulges posterior/inferiorly with visualization of the cystocele.

13. 11–1 OC

14. Yes, it is elevated toward the defect.

15. There is markedly increased vascularity along the mid to left lateral aspect of the ASC, indicating inflammation of this area.

16. a. It is placed *on* the residual sling that appears to be located at the anterior central (mid) and to left lateral vaginal wall, best seen on the initial and rotated C plane (screen bottom images, Fig. 251).
    b. Mid, which is best seen on the A plane
    c. Mid to left
    The 3D rendered image (Fig. 252) clearly demonstrates continued presence of nearly the entire sling, except at the lateral right arm.

17. The secondary hypoechoic area (gold arrow) is posterior and inferior to the bladder.

18. b (with progressive urinoma visualized beyond tract)

19. The normal vaginal length is approximately 8–9 cm.

20. The vagina is markedly shortened and curved on this patient. The measurement was traced at 3.99 cm.

21. a. Bladder
    b. Symphysis pubis
    c. Urethra
    d. Vagina
    e. Inferior
    f. Posterior
    g. Superior
    h. Anterior

22. Mid-distal

23. a. A is sagittal of the urethra (and sagittal to the body)
    b. B is coronal of the posterior urethra (and coronal to the body)
    c. C is transverse of the urethra (and transverse to the body)

24. a

25. The distance is 1.1 cm.

26. Note on the Fig. 267 description that relationships of structures and relative echo patterns are emphasized. The reader should be able to imagine from the description how the findings appear.

27. The measurement is 2.2 × 2.3 cm. It should be reported that the shape is trapezoidal with a mid- to high-level heterogeneous echo pattern.

28. The B plane does not demonstrate it at all because the B plane is a coronal cut of the urethra in front of the sling. The A and B planes best differentiates the bladder wall/fascial sling interface. The gold arrows point to the urethral wall and the blue arrows point to the fascial sling border.

29. Since it is subjective, any answer comparing the 3D quality with 2D quality is correct.

30. a. It is placed on the mid-urethral mucosa, slightly left of ML.
    b. It is empty, as seen on the ML sagittal A plane of the volume set (gold arrow).

31. d. Though there is an acoustic shadowing beyond the air in the rectum, it is not the reason for the increased echo pattern.

32. Yes, it is intact with no elevation of the central mucosa.

33. Color Power Doppler indicates a focal area of slightly increased vascularity likely from past inflammation of this area, now healed and consistent with her delivery history.

34. The transducer can be rotated 90 degrees to stretch out the structure as in the 2D image on Fig. 276 if 3D imaging is not available or only 2D

EV imaging is being done. Note the CRP on all the 3D volume set images and how its placement near the stitch with presence of surrounding bladder urine brings the 3D rendered image of the elongated stitch into clear view as seen on Fig. 277. Findings are consistent with an aberrantly placed surgical stitch.

35. b. The green arrow well-delineates the fistula tracking. On real time, the air may appear to "gurgle" from posterior to anterior. The blue arrow clarifies where the fistula tracking take-off occurs at the 12 OC IAS. Post-processing chroma is a tool that alters the acquired image by manipulating the image color hue. On this example of a rectovaginal fistula, chroma post-processing, used on the right, subjectively crisps up borders of the air going through the fistula tracking from the anal sphincter through the vaginal wall. Fortunately, multiple chroma options are variable and can be altered after an image is frozen at a workstation screen.

Chapter 8: Case Reviews 129–150

2. b. The ovary is comprised of a large well-circumscribed smooth-walled mass, measuring $10 \times 6 \times 5.2$ cm.

3. a. The echo pattern is complex, primarily cystic in appearance with a vertical septum along the superior right of ML aspect of the lesion around which there are two clusters of hyperechoic spherical papillations noted, ranging in size from approximately 4mm to 6 mm in diameter. Your sonographic DDx would include borderline mucinous tumor, mucinous cystadenoma, mucinous cystadenocarcinoma, and serous cystadenoma as well as other malignant neoplasms. The ultimate diagnosis is from microscopic pathologic assessment. In this case, the pathologic diagnosis was a papillomatous mucinous cystadenocarcinoma.

4. a. No
   b. No
   c. Yes
   d. Yes
   e. Yes

5. a (gold arrows); b (green arrows). The anteverted uterus demonstrates a bulbous appearance with a heterogeneous echo pattern, especially at the fundal right endometrial/myometrial interface, where the border is poorly seen and is adjacent to a cluster of diffuse very small hypoechoic lesions measuring 1–2 mm. Additionally, the myometrium contains several round but poorly circumscribed myomatous lesions along the posterior intramural uterine segment. Color Power Doppler elicits a paucity of vascularity around the fundal endometrium. Findings are consistent with adenomyosis. It is not unusual to find concomitant leiomyomata, as is the case here, for studies have shown that up to about 40% of cases have both.

6. One large line to another represents 5 cm. One small line to another represents 1 cm and one small line to a dot represents 0.5 cm. This mass measures approximately $5.1 \times 5.05 \times 6.2$ cm with a volume of 83.03 cm^3 using the prolate ellipsoid volume formula and the irregular hyperechoic mural wall lesion measures $1.67 \times 2.85 \times 2.15$ cm with a volume of 5.3 cm^3.

7. The resistive index is the most commonly utilized formula, calculated by subtracting the end-diastolic velocity (EDV) from the peak systolic velocity (PSV) and divided by the PSV. The RI will be automatically calculated by the ultrasound system when calipers are placed on the peak systole and end diastole on the waveform. The normal ovarian flow RI typically measures > 0.4. Suspicion for malignancy is increased when the RI is below 0.4 within an ovarian mass. A quickly developing vessel formation in a malignant neoplasm is theorized to occur with reduced integrity of the normal elastic recoil in systole of the last-to-form middle layer (as opposed to the intima and adventitia layers). This lack of flow resistance results in increased peak diastolic flow, leading to a reduced RI. Note that in this case, the RI is particularly low at 0.2. As can be seen in this spectral flow pattern, when the peak flows of both diastole and systole get closer to each other, it may be difficult to even differentiate the peak and end points on the spectral waveform. Histologic diagnosis of this mass was a serous cystadenocarcinoma.

8. a. Yes
   b. No, it is circumferentially intact.
   c. No, it is central.
   d. It is at the midlevel because of visualization of the PVM complex (white arrows).

9. c. The level of the transducer through the cuff is important to appreciate, as the cuff may appear normal in contour at one level like this image, but an abnormality could be missed at just a slightly different level; so, like any general survey of the anatomy at the beginning of any exam, in the absence of a uterus on a patient with pain, sweep through the cuff anteriorly to posteriorly in the transverse plane and lateral to lateral in a sagittal plane while noting the contour. The sagittal image (screen bottom) shows arbitrary cuts (green lines) at different levels than the centered abnormal finding, where the cuff would have appeared normal. In this case, the white lines overlie the left ovary which is located directly superior/adjacent to the cuff. The interface is also adjacent to bowel and distorted cuff contour (red arrows). The examiner's lower abdominal palpation of the opposite hand toward the transducer while imaging the ovary did not separate or alter the contour, making it likely that the ovary is adhered to the cuff and a reasonable etiology for continued pain. The presence of a small endometrial implant at this interface cannot be excluded.

10. a. It appears contiguous with the myometrium (yellow arrows).
    b. It appears mostly isoechoic as related to the uterus, although is diffusely heterogeneous with evident sound absorption from the initial aspect to distal aspect of mass.

11. a. No
    b. No
    Neither appears part of the mass. The right ovary is well seen as separate from the uterus. Though the left ovary is displaced to the far-left aspect of the pelvis by the mass, it is distinctly separate, as well. Several images demonstrate contiguity to the intrauterine gestation with the uterine cavity; therefore, the mass appears uterine in origin.

12. Fig. 288 demonstrates the calipers at $13.54 \times 9.19 \times 12.06$ cm with a volume of 785.7 cm^3, calculated by using the prolate ellipsoid volume formula and measuring $L \times W \times H \times 0.52$.

13. b

14. Neither the number nor size raises concern. It is typical to see several nabothian cysts on the normal gynecologic examination; however, it

is not of concern when this many are present.

15. Color Power Doppler
16. b
17. b (middle gold arrow)
18. A is the patient's right.
19. b. "Stretching out" the contiguous anechoic fold of the 3D rendered structure that appears folded over itself confirms a sonographic diagnosis of hydrosalpinx.
20. The arrows are pointing to para-uterine intraperitoneal free fluid.
21. c
22. b. Surgical pathology diagnosis was a hemorrhagic corpus luteum.
23. a and d. By merely magnifying the image (turning the zoom or magnification knob), the examiner will effectively just make bigger pixels as the image appears bigger, while not improving the image resolution. This is referred to as "read zoom." "Write zoom" occurs by pushing the zoom knob and bringing up the zoom box onto the screen, which is telling the ultrasound system that you want to make the image magnified but not the whole image, and that you are going to purposely place a box around what is to be zoomed. By narrowing the magnifying box to the area of interest and pushing the zoom knob again, the lines of site within the box will be closer together when rewritten ("write" zoomed) and the new image will have a higher frame rate (FR), which is the number of times per second a new image is changed; thus, improving the resolution. Fig. 302 demonstrates a frame rate (FR) of 50 frames per second (seen at the top left as 50 Hertz (Hz). The improved resolution of Fig. 303, however, is apparent, and the annotated FR is 130 Hz. Sometimes when learning a new ultrasound system, the "FR" label on the control screen can be confused with "frequency."
24. d. The homogeneous echo pattern of the overall endometrium comprises the now thickened functional layer that appears more echogenic as it becomes denser. This results in an echo pattern that is more like (isoechoic) that of the basal layer, measuring about 16 mm.
25. a. The Doppler RI was under the 0.40 threshold of normal. Because of the persistent heterogeneity of the ovary, the patient was taken to

surgery. The pathologic diagnosis was multiple follicular cysts.
26. With a symmetric smooth-walled appearance of the pubovisceralis muscle (PVM) complex, there appears to be no evidence of lateral avulsion injury noted. Rotation of the anterior plane would have enhanced complete visualization of the PVM complex/symphysis attachment.
27. b. Though all the first few calipers are not shown on the screen, the 5 and 10 cm distances are, so depth can be noted. Each dot along the right side of the image is 1 cm. Each horizontal line is 5 cm.
28. b. Pathology at surgery indicated this as a malignant neoplasm.
29. "Have you had a cesarean section?" Sharp anterior extension of the cavity is clearly seen at the LUS, enhanced with residual infused fluid for the sonohysterogram procedure.
30. a. Yes
    b. No, it is nearly empty.
    c. No, it is at the mid-urethra.
    d. Yes
    e. Yes
31. C plane
32. Distal. In fact, the distance from the sling to the perineal surface is 5 mm (yellow line); therefore, it is not supporting the urethra.
33. a. The frame rate is 7 Hz (red arrow).
    d. This image is Color Power Doppler which is a qualitative representation of vascularity within the uterus and endometrium, providing a global image of where the vessels are.
    c. The frequency of the EV transducer is 5–9 MHz and the exam pre-settings are "GYN" (gold arrow).
    d. The large-to-large horizontal calipers along the left side of the screen represent 5 cm, but the image has been read zoomed (magnified), so the first horizontal caliper is not seen; therefore, another place to check the depth of view is also under the transducer frequency in this case, which is 8.9 cm of depth, or field of view (green arrow). The middle number below the transducer information at the top of the image is the amount the image has been magnified, which is 1.9x (blue arrow).

34. a. Transperineal
    b. Yes
    c. No
    d. Yes
    e. Yes
    f. B
35. Both
36. A
37. Mid-urethra

Chapter 9: Case Reviews 151–165

2. a. The urethra is bulky in appearance with an irregular contour and thickened wall.
   b. There appears to be partial residual mesh with several linear echogenic foci and thickening noted along the mid to right posterior aspect of the urethra (yellow arrow).
   c. Though seen posterior to the urethra, it is more thickened along the mid to right side.
3. It is seen at the proximal urethral level at the cross section of the orthogonal planes. It should be at the mid-urethral level to be the most effective in urethral support.
4. c
5. The mesh is asymmetric with thickened hyperechoic foci noted along the posterior aspect; therefore, very little mesh appears to have been resected.
6. a
7. a. The basal (gold arrows), functional (red arrows), and central cavity (green arrow) layers are distinct; however, the functional layer is not thickened, as it recently sloughed off.
8. b
9. d. The sonographic differential diagnosis (DDx) would include a hemorrhagic corpus luteum for this type of appearance, especially with the peripheral flow around the smaller central lesion, as it appears to have resolved by half in size and a changed central echo pattern. There is minimal free fluid noted in the PCDS (Fig. 322, blue arrow), which would not be uncommon with a ruptured cyst. The RI is increased, though we do not know the previous RI. A resolving corpus luteum would likely have originally been lower; however, as it heals, the RI will rise as it has at the current exam. Depending on whether there continues to be clinical symptoms, one more follow-up exam in 8 weeks would likely demonstrate complete resolution. To do another

expensive exam too soon, however, with possible incomplete resolution, the desired normal appearance may not yet have occurred. The exam was repeated 7 weeks later, and the lesion and free fluid were completely resolved, confirming the likelihood of a resolved hemorrhagic corpus luteum.

10. Retroverted
11. d. The thickened endometrium is globally homogeneous in echo pattern wherein the functional and basal layers are typically isoechoic.
12. Intraendometrial
13. c. The green arrows point to bilateral tortuous dilated uterine vascularity, suggestive of pelvic congestion.
14. There is no concentric peripheral flow around the lesion as there would be around a gestational sac where it would represent vascular perigestational sac trophoblast.
15. c
16. a (though the flexion is slight)
17. Orthogonal planes are straight lines relative to the CRP. The IUD is not seen because with the slight retroflexion, the endometrial cavity at the midlevel where the stem would be more anterior than the CRP location and arms, as indicated by the gold line, so is not seen on any orthogonal plane.
18. 1. Acoustic shadow of the IUD. The IUD stem is hyperechoic as related to the hypoechoic shadow and is not seen because it is anterior to this slice.
    2. IUD string. This is seen as hyperechoic because the ultrasound lines of sight are hitting the strings perpendicularly.
    3. Ovary. Whether it is the left or right ovary is undetectable until the CRP is moved to the ovary on the A plane, at which time the ovarian location will be seen on all three planes. There is an oval-shaped anechoic subcomponent seen, consistent with a follicle or corpus luteum.
19. Using the prolate ellipsoid formula, the uterine volume calculation is $10.51 \times 8.27 \times 9.5 \times 0.52 = $ **429.4 cm³**, far exceeding the typical 56 cm³ postmenopausal uterus.
20. a
21. The 2-cm circular hyperechoic structure represents a common intrauterine device (IUD) used in China, the stainless-steel Shanghai ring IUD (Fig. 337a). It is located at the lower left endometrium.
22. c. The arrow is pointing to free fluid within the posterior cul-de-sac, indicating the patency of at least one of the fallopian tubes.
23. a. The basal layer is the only layer seen (gold arrow).
24. c. The endometrial cavity contains a small amount of free fluid creating somewhat a self-induced sonohysterogram that surrounds an echogenic cluster of intracavitary lesions that are isoechoic to the endometrium.
25. It is isoechoic relative to the endometrium.
26. It is irregular and multilobulated.
27. c
28. Endometrial polyps
29. d
30. The A component has the appearance of recent acute hemorrhage, whereas B demonstrates an irregular heterogeneous complex primarily solid appearance within a rim of an irregular luminal wall thickness. Final surgical pathology indicated this was a borderline tumor.
31. Yes
32. Both. Within the lower uterine segment (LUS) there is a small circle of slightly hyperechoic interfaces present. By post-processing the Fig. 343 image to highlight contrast, Fig. 344 enhances the presence of that small cluster of echoes, localizing the strings at the LUS (gold arrows). So, all demonstrate the strings and post-processing the image on Fig. 344 accentuates the strings.
33. b
34. c. The high-contrast 2D image (screen right, Fig. 346) demonstrates a heterogeneous endometrial echo pattern that the smooth 3D image did not visualize. Additionally, abnormal endometrial vascularity within the lesions is noted. While the original endometrial 3D volume set appears symmetrically homogeneous and increased in thickness, which is consistent with the patient's secretory phase menstrual history, application of Color Power Doppler demonstrating abnormal vascularity into the endometrium plus the more heterogeneous echo pattern with post-processing, several small round hyperechoic lesions are noted, findings consistent with endometrial polyps.

35. a. 119 frames per second (FR)
    b. Write zoomed after a narrow zoom box magnification was placed over an original image, resulting in increased resolution
    c. 12–3 o'clock (OC)
    d. Yes
    e. Pubovisceralis muscle (PVM) complex
    f. Mid IAS
36. b
37. Even though the myoma is nearly the size of the uterus, it does not lie close enough to alter the endometrial contour, which remains smooth. Additionally, it is unlikely the etiology for the patient's menorrhagia.
38. b
39. a
40. f
41. c. The patient underwent a bilateral salpingo-oophorectomy (BSO) and pathology revealed a borderline tumor.
42. No. The mesh is seen at the anterior vaginal wall and the extending lateral aspects are well visualized; however, at what urethral segment these cuts are made cannot be determined unless a ML sagittal image is done.
43. b
44. d
45. It is supported.

Chapter 10: Case Reviews 166–184

2. a. Yes, and it is best seen on the A and C planes and the rendered image.
   b. Yes, and they are only seen on the C plane and the rendered image.
   c. No, it is anteverted.
   d. Yes, it is brought down *to* the IUD on the A plane.
   e. It is located at the cross point between the arms and the stem and can be seen on all planes (gold arrows). The IUD stem is not seen because the CRP cuts the sagittal plane below the stem location (white line).
   f. Yes
   g. They are pointing to the IUD string.
3. a. If the CRP is placed where the IUD is not present, it is simply out of the chosen plane, which is why the stem is not visualized. It is, however, in the volume set and could be found by parallel shifting through the volume.

4. b. The C plane image has been rotated upright on the Z-axis to more intuitively view the IUD (bottom screen right). The arms are positioned at the fundal end of the cavity and extend into the myometrium (abnormal). The stem is likely within the cavity; however, the stem is not seen because the orthogonal planes are off plane by misplacement of the CRP on the volume set. The examiner could move the CRP to the arms and then move anteriorly to posteriorly through the uterus until the stem comes into view or the examiner could parallel shift through the rendered image until the stem comes into view to refine the assessment.

5. a. Left
   b. Right
   c. Left
   d. Right

6. At the hilum. Note that while the 2D Color Power Doppler demonstrates increased flow, the profound cumulative 3D color power image (Fig. 365) is better appreciated, increasing the suspicion for morbidity.

7. b. Diagnosis at pathology was a dysgerminoma.

8. b. There is a distinct indentation of the anterior wall of the uterus at the LUS, underneath which there is a hypoechoic elongated area that is contiguous with the elevated hyperechoic endometrium into the hypoechoic area. This is not a uterine anomaly because this is at the LUS only. Findings are consistent with a cesarean section scar.

9. b The A sweep plane is sagittal.

10. c. The CRP on this image is pale yellow on the A plane, red on the B plane, and pale blue on the C plane.

11. No. Normally, the AP diameter is not measured but subjectively consistent from inferior to superior. The AP diameter measures progressively smaller from proximal to distal, at 15.5, 14.5, and 8.2 mm, theoretically from compression of the rectal prolapse (posterior to the vagina).

12. a. This oval-shaped folded extension originates at the distal anterior internal sphincter and measures approximately 13 × 18 mm. The 3D rendered image demonstrates only the anterior hypoechoic aspect of the prolapse. The concave appearing anal curve noted on a midsagittal cut through the pelvic floor is typically smooth in contour with no alteration of the vaginal canal symmetry anterior to it. Findings are consistent with a rectal prolapse.

13. b. There are marked diffuse trabeculations from long-term consequences associated with spina bifida and persistent urine stasis and self-catheterization.

14. d.

15. PVR is calculated by measuring the length × width × height × 0.52 (prolate ellipsoid formula for volume measurement). Calipers are seen along the side of the image and can be used to measure volume post exam. A PVR < 100 mL is considered normal. A PVR of 100–200 mL is not normal, but not necessarily of clinical significance and a PVR > 200 mL should be worked up. This PVR is normal at 38.6 cm³.

16. a

17. b. Note that several intramural myomatous lesions are present, all of which demonstrate the same heterogeneous echo pattern, and that this lesion creates a posterior acoustic shadow indicating a dense structure; therefore, of these differentials, the most likely would be a submucosal myoma.

18. Sagittal. 3D transperineal volume sets of the pelvic floor in this workbook will all be with a midsagittal sweep plane. The sagittal A plane of the urethra will also be the body plane.

19. Coronal

20. Axial

21. c. The blue arrows are pointing to the sling as if looking into it on the A plane and transverse view from behind on the C plane. While the C plane most obviously demonstrates the presence of the suburethral sling, the C plane by itself, however, does not demonstrate if it is at the appropriate level. To establish the level (proximal, mid, or distal), the A (sagittal) plane must be assessed and included in the imaging record. In this case, the sling is seen at the correct mid-level.

22. a. A as evidenced by the pixel blush
    b. D as evidenced by normal flow and very mild blush
    c. B as evidenced by diffuse lack of vascular flow
    d. C as evidenced by normal vessel distribution

23. a. The calipers are along the side of the image. The typical thickness of a postmenopausal woman is 2–3 mm, but normal endometrial thickness is considered less than 5 mm.

24. c. The uterine artery branches to the arcuate arteries, which travel along the uterine periphery (parallel to the endometrium), and branch to the radial arteries, which travel perpendicularly through the myometrium, which branch to become the smallest spiral arteries lying perpendicular to without crossing the endometrium.

25. d. The green arrow is the patient's left. Findings are consistent with a rectovaginal fistula tracking toward the vagina.

26. Fig. 387 measures the right ovarian mass at 10.72 × 9.93 × 7.72 cm with a volume of 430 cm³; therefore, it is markedly enlarged.

27. d

28. a. Anterior
    b. To the patient's right

29. c

30. b and e

31. It is pointing to the IUD string within the cervical canal.

32. d

33. The IAS is contiguous through the trace, proving the IAS is folded over itself and consistent with a rectocele.

34. a. Cervical homogeneity is the normal appearance.

35. a and c

36. No

37. Heterogeneous with low-level echoes and diffuse punctate echogenic foci

38. No

39. c

Index

Page numbers followed by "*f*" indicate figures